MEDITARRANEAN COOKBOOK FOR PREGANT WOMEN

120 PLUS DELICIOUS DIET WITH PICTURES

BY

MAXWELL JOE

Copyright@ MAXWELL JOE 2024

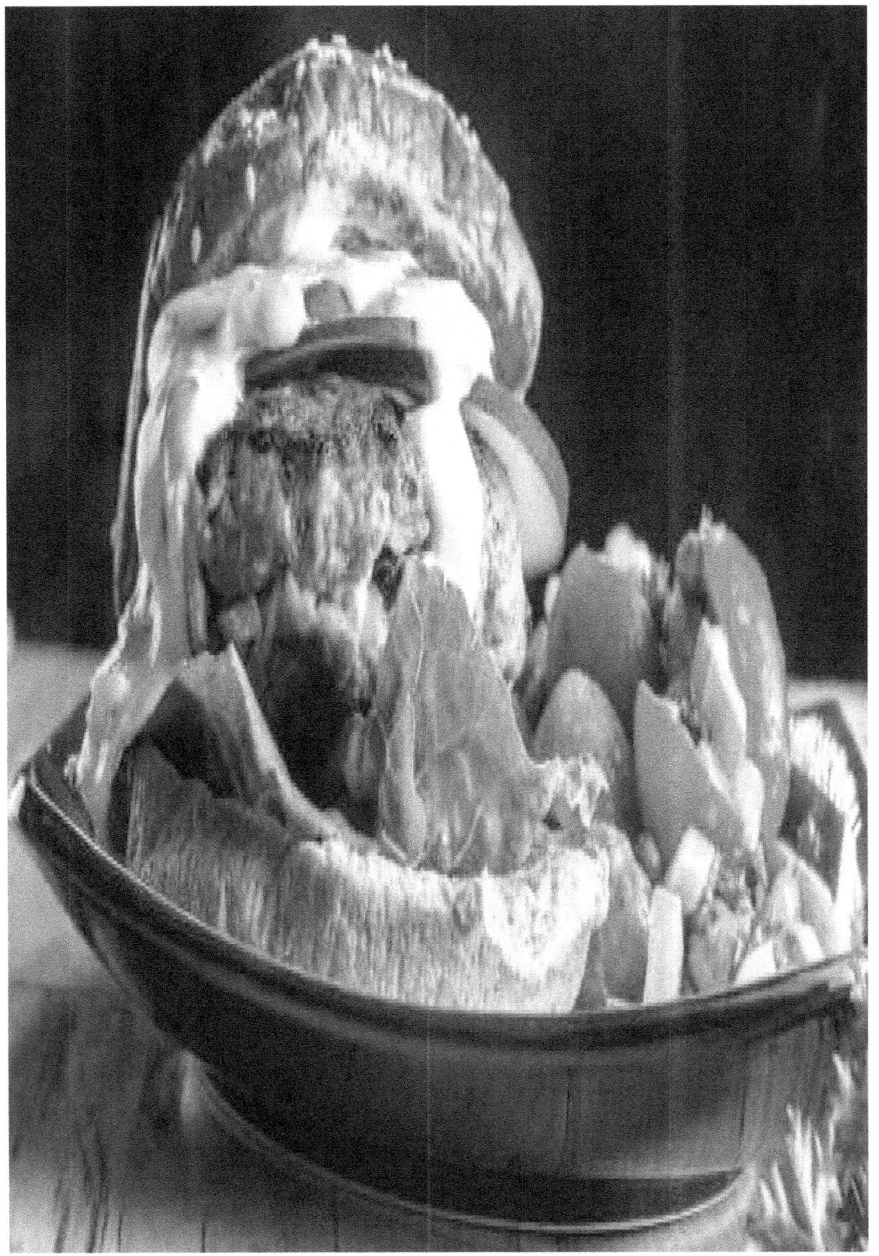

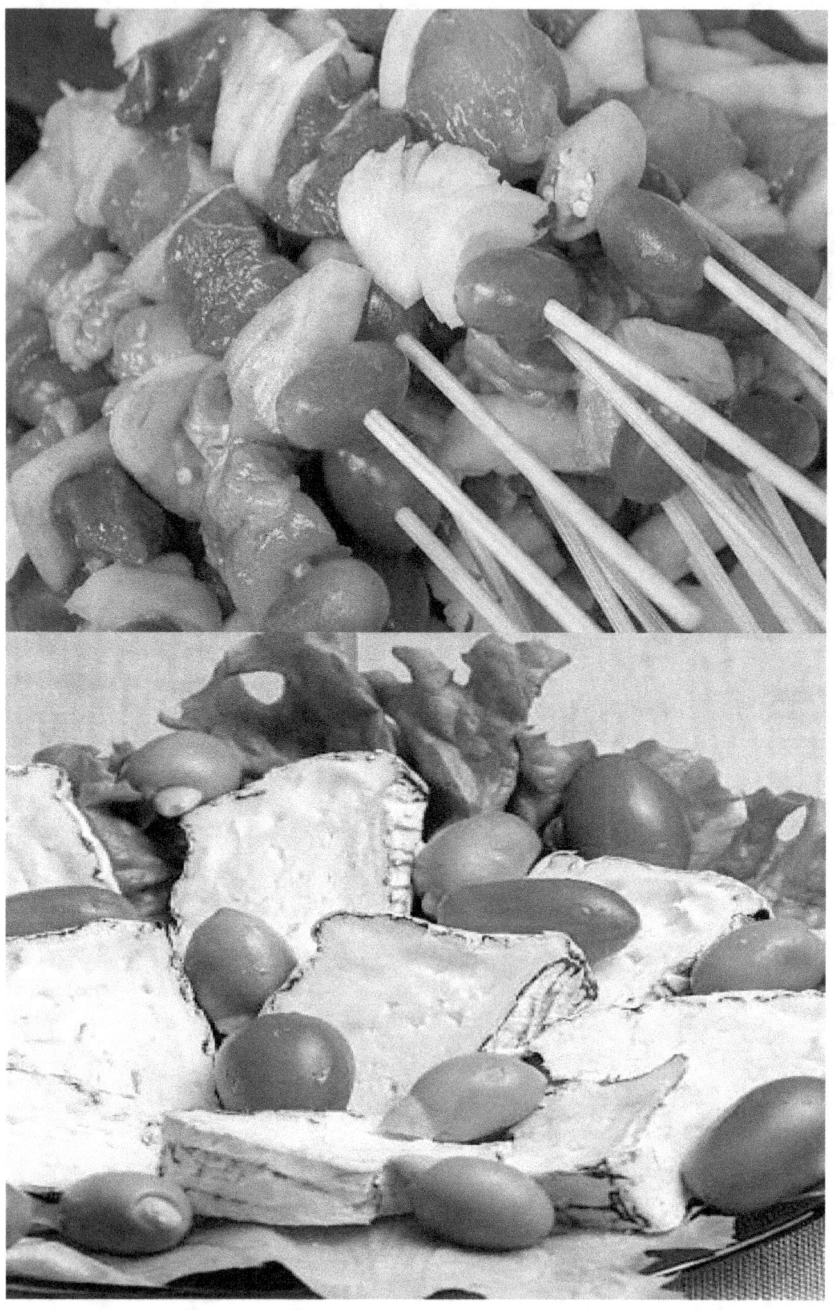

ABOUT THE AUTHOR

MAXWELL JOE is someone that believes that knowledge is power, the more you acquire it, the more chances you get.

TABLE OF CONTENTS

DESCRIPTION

"The Mediterranean Diet Cookbook for Pregnant women" This cookbook provides a broad range of alternatives for breakfast, lunch, supper, snacks, and even desserts with over 120 delicious dishes. This book has something for everyone, from colorful salads and filling soups to tasty seafood recipes and filling vegetarian dinners. However, it goes beyond the recipes. We also provide you useful advice on how to apply the Mediterranean lifestyle to your everyday activities. Learn how to shop for groceries and plan meals so you can easily make healthy choices. "The Mediterranean Diet Cookbook for pregnant women" is the ideal travel companion for anybody looking to adopt a healthier pregnancy, regardless of experience level with the diet. Making nutritious meals has never been more fun thanks to the clear directions and gorgeous photos that go with each dish. Embrace the Mediterranean recipes and experience the life-changing benefits it has brought to millions of people's health and wellbeing. Are you prepared to travel the Mediterranean with your taste buds? Get a copy of this book right now to begin satisfying your palate and nourishing your body.

CHAPTER ONE

Understanding the Mediterranean Diet

The many health advantages of the Mediterranean diet, especially its favorable effects on pregnancy and mother health, have won it international recognition. Adopting a Mediterranean diet may be very beneficial for expectant mothers since it offers a nutrient-rich, balanced eating plan that promotes the mother's health as well as the health of the growing child.

The Mediterranean Diet's Advantages for Expectant Mothers

1. **Rich in elements**: Vitamins, minerals, and antioxidants are just a few of the vital elements that are plentiful in the Mediterranean diet and are important for a healthy pregnancy. These nutrients enhance the health of the mother overall, boost fetal growth, and lower the chance of birth abnormalities.

2. **Heart Health**: The heart-healthy elements of the Mediterranean diet, such as almonds, olive oil, and fatty fish, are well-known. Eating these foods during pregnancy may help reduce the risk of preeclampsia and gestational hypertension, two frequent pregnancy problems.

3. **Weight management**: Pregnant women who adhere to the Mediterranean diet are more likely to maintain a healthy weight during their pregnancy. Prioritizing healthy meals, fruits, vegetables, and lean meats will help minimize the risk of issues like gestational diabetes and avoid excessive weight gain.

4. **Decreased Inflammation**: The Mediterranean diet's anti-inflammatory qualities might help reduce pregnancy-related discomforts such joint pain and edema. Expectant mothers may benefit from increased comfort and mobility during their pregnancy by decreasing inflammation in the body.

5. **Better Digestion**: The Mediterranean diet's high fiber content, which comes from whole grains, legumes, fruits, and vegetables, may help maintain a healthy digestive system and fend against typical pregnancy-related problems like constipation.

<u>Important Elements of a Mediterranean Diet</u>

1. **Plant-Based Foods**: Fruits, vegetables, whole grains, legumes, nuts, and seeds are among the plant-based foods that form the basis of the Mediterranean diet. Essential nutrients, fiber, and antioxidants included in these meals promote general health and wellbeing.

2. **Healthful Fats**: The main source of fat in a Mediterranean diet is olive oil, which is a mainstay. Olive oil, which is high in monounsaturated fats and antioxidants, supports heart health, lowers inflammation, and fosters a baby's normal development of the brain.

3. **Lean Proteins**: Fish, poultry, and lentils are among the moderately high-lean protein foods included in the Mediterranean diet. These protein sources include vital minerals like iron and omega-3 fatty acids and are crucial for the growth and development of the fetus.

4. **Dairy items**: The Mediterranean diet calls for

moderation when it comes to dairy items like cheese and Greek yogurt. These protein and calcium sources help maintain the mother's and the unborn child's healthy bones during pregnancy.

5. **Herbs and Spices**: Mediterranean cooking makes extensive use of herbs and spices to enhance taste without resorting to too much sugar or salt. Herbs that give extra antioxidants and nutritional benefits to food, such as oregano, basil, and thyme, also improve its flavor.

6. **Moderate Wine intake**: If you're not pregnant, you should still abstain from alcohol, but moderate wine intake is a traditional part of the Mediterranean diet for everyone else. However, in order to protect their unborn child's health and wellbeing, expectant mothers should abstain from alcohol throughout their pregnancy.

Including these essential elements of the Mediterranean diet in your regular meals will help provide a strong basis for a happy and healthy pregnancy. Expecting mothers may enhance their well-being during this unique period by prioritizing nutrient-dense foods, well-balanced meals, and mindful eating practices.

CHAPTER TWO

Crucial Elements for a Fit Pregnancy

One of the most crucial components of being ready for this trip is making sure your body is well-nourished with critical nutrients. Being ready for pregnancy is an exciting and significant period in a woman's life. In addition to supporting your general health, a well-balanced, high-nutrient diet may increase your chances of becoming pregnant and delivering a safe and healthy baby. Let's talk about the foods you can eat to increase your fertility and the important nutrients for a healthy pregnancy.

Crucial Elements for a Fit Pregnancy:

1. **Folic Acid**: Also referred to as folate, folic acid is a B vitamin that is essential for avoiding neural tube abnormalities in growing infants. To lower their

chance of birth abnormalities, women of reproductive age should take 400–800 mcg of folic acid every day. Citrus fruits, legumes, fortified cereals, and leafy green vegetables are good dietary sources of folic acid.

2. **Iron**: Iron is necessary for the synthesis of hemoglobin, which transports oxygen to your body's cells and the developing fetus. Your body requires more iron during pregnancy in order to support the placenta's growth and blood volume expansion. Lean meats, chicken, fish, beans, lentils, and fortified cereals are good sources of iron.

3. **Calcium:** Your baby's teeth, muscles, and bones all grow with the help of calcium. Additionally, it supports your baby's and your own good blood pressure and muscular performance. Rich sources of calcium include leafy green vegetables, almonds, and fortified plant-based milks, as well as dairy products like milk, yogurt, and cheese.

4. **Omega-3 Fatty Acids**: Your baby's brain and vision are developing because of omega-3 fatty acids, especially DHA (docosahexaenoic acid). They may also help lower the risk of premature delivery and

promote the mental health of mothers. Omega-3s are abundant in fatty fish, walnuts, chia seeds, and flaxseeds, as well as in walnuts, sardines, and mackerel.

5. **Protein:** You and your unborn child's tissues need on protein for development and repair. It also affects immunological response and hormone synthesis. Lean meats, poultry, fish, eggs, dairy products, legumes, nuts, and seeds are all excellent sources of protein.

CHAPTER THREE

Nourishing Breakfast Recipes

1. Greek Yogurt Parfait

Prep Time: 5 minutes

Ingredients: Greek yogurt, honey, granola, mixed berries

Method:

1. In a bowl, layer Greek yogurt, honey, granola, and mixed berries.

2.Redo the layers and enjoy.

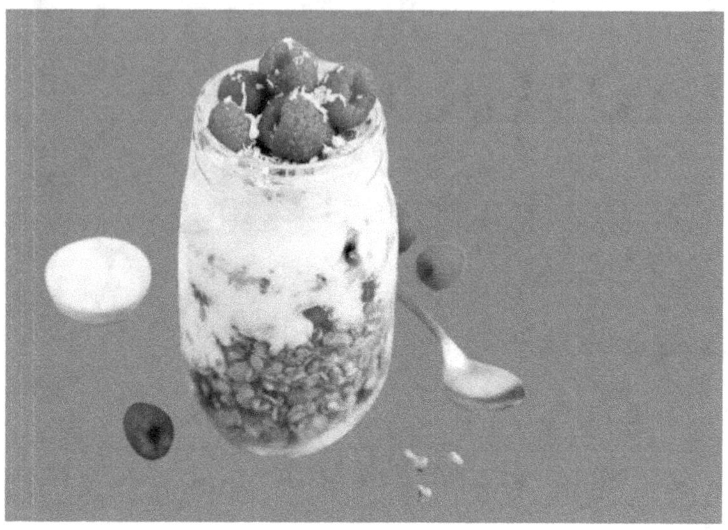

2. <u>Shakshuka</u>

Prep Time: 20 minutes

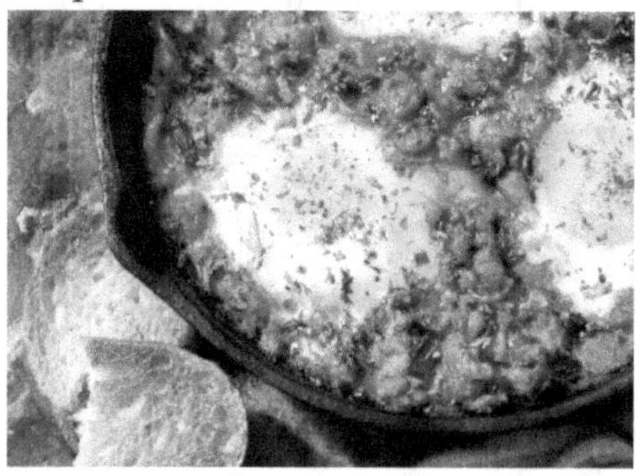

Ingredients: Eggs, tomatoes, bell peppers, onions, garlic, cumin, paprika, feta cheese

Method:

1. Sauté onions, bell peppers, and garlic in a pan.
2. Add tomatoes, cumin, and paprika.
3. Break eggs into the mixture and cook until the eggs are
   set.
4. Top with crumbled feta cheese.Enjoy!

3. <u>**Mediterranean Veggie Omelette**</u>

Prep Time: 15 minutes

Ingredients: Eggs, bell peppers, tomatoes, spinach, feta cheese, olives

Method:

1. Whisk eggs and pour into a pan.
2. Add chopped bell peppers, tomatoes, spinach, feta cheese, and olives.
3. Cook until the eggs are ready.

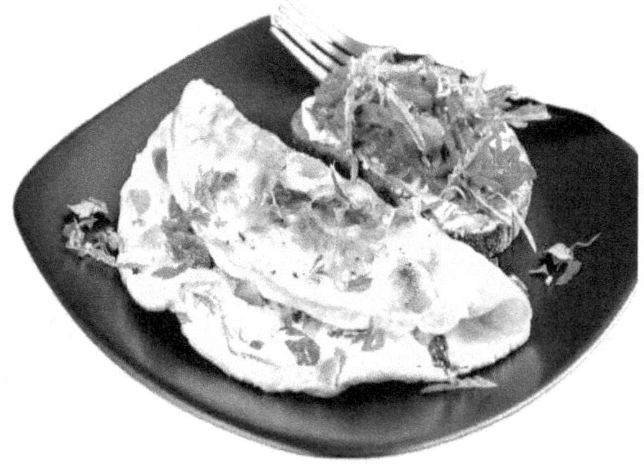

4. <u>**Avocado Toast with Poached Eggs**</u>

Prep Time: 10 minutes

Ingredients: Whole grain bread, avocado, poached eggs, cherry tomatoes, arugula

Method:

1. Toast bread and top with mashed avocado.
2. Place poached eggs on top and garnish with cherry tomatoes and arugula, Enjoy!

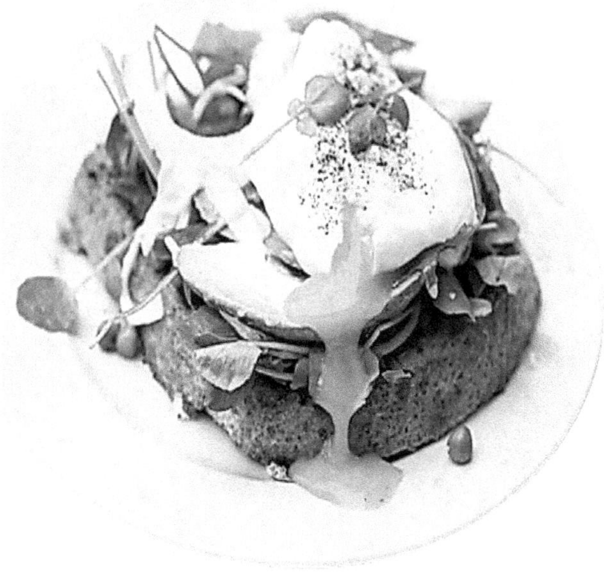

5. <u>Mediterranean Quinoa Breakfast Bowl</u>

Prep Time: 20 minutes

Ingredients: Quinoa, cucumber, cherry tomatoes, olives, feta cheese, lemon juice

Method:

1. Cook quinoa according to package instructions. Mix in chopped cucumber, cherry tomatoes, olives, feta cheese
2. Squeeze of lemon juice, it is yummy!

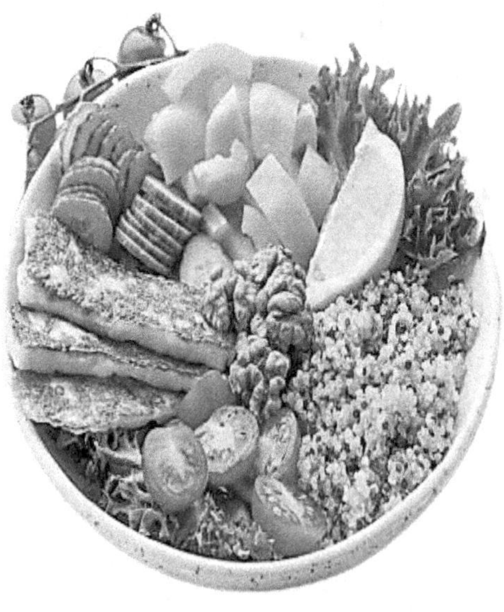

6. **<u>Spinach and Feta Frittata</u>**

Prep Time: 25 minutes

Ingredients: Eggs, spinach, feta cheese, onions, garlic

Method:

1. Sauté onions and garlic in a pan.
2. Add spinach and cook until wilted.
3. Pour whisked eggs over the mixture and top with crumbled feta cheese.
4. Bake until set.

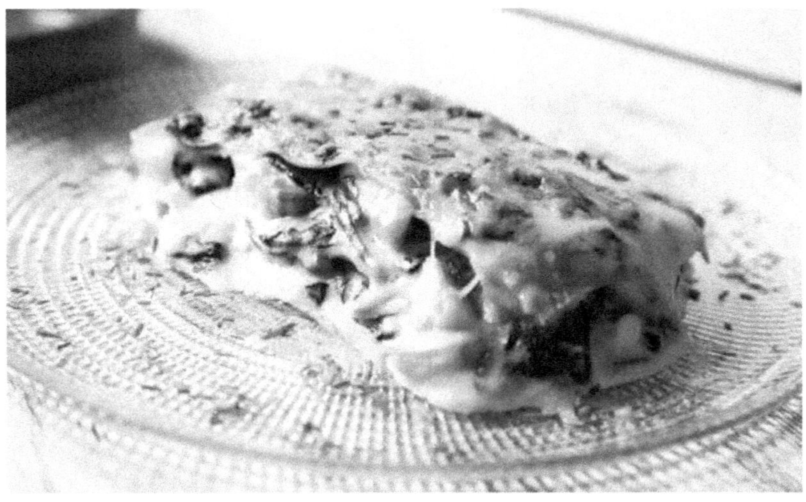

7. **<u>Mediterranean Breakfast Burrito</u>**

Prep Time: 15 minutes

Ingredients: Whole wheat tortilla, scrambled eggs, roasted red peppers, feta cheese, olives

Method:

1. Fill a tortilla with scrambled eggs, roasted red peppers, crumbled feta cheese, and sliced olives.
2. Roll up and enjoy.

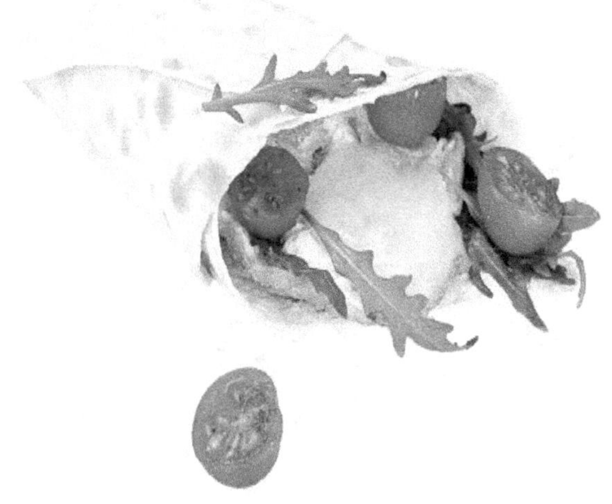

8. <u>Lemon Blueberry Overnight Oats</u>

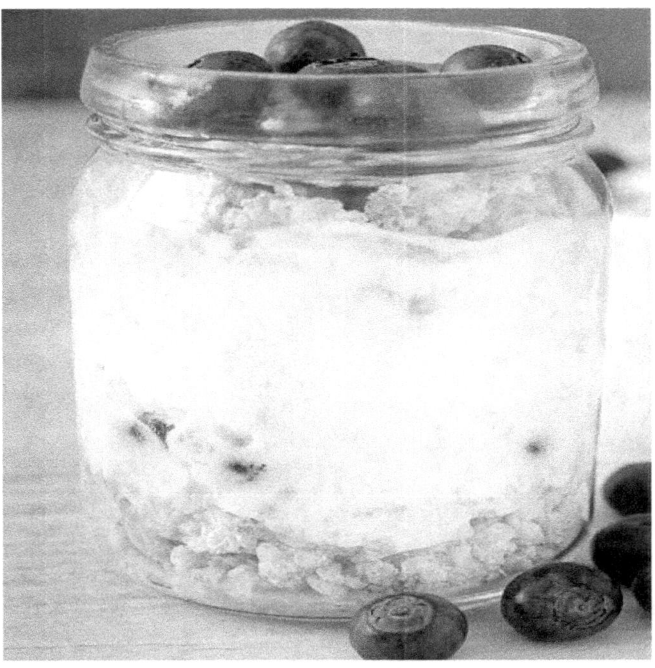

Prep Time: 5 minutes (plus overnight soaking)

Ingredients: Rolled oats, almond milk, lemon zest, blueberries, honey

Method: Mix oats with almond milk, lemon zest, blueberries, and honey in a jar. Let it sit in thefridge overnight.

9. **<u>Mediterranean Breakfast Skewers</u>**

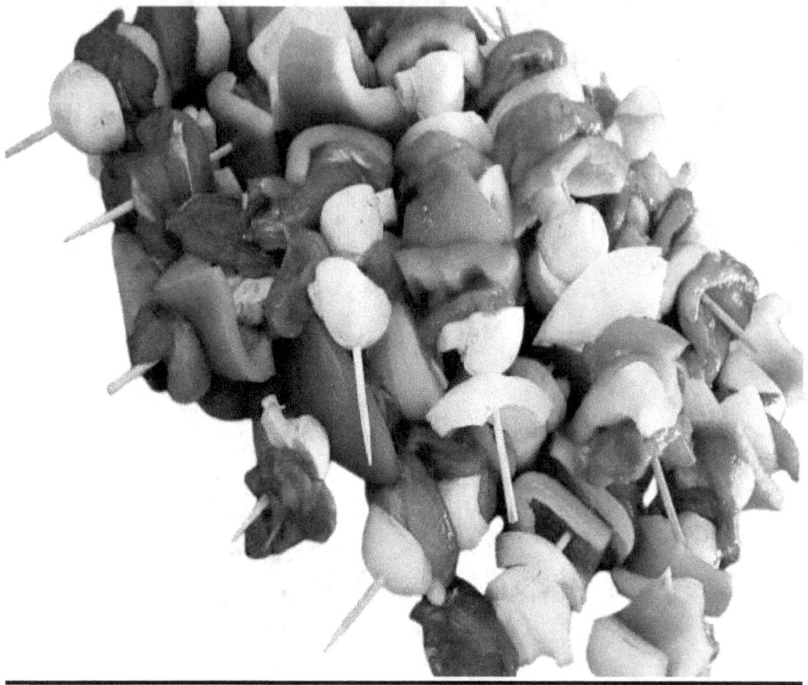

Prep Time: 10 minutes

Ingredients: Cherry tomatoes, cucumber slices, olives, feta cheese cubes

Method: Thread cherry tomatoes, cucumber slices, olives, and feta cheese cubes onto skewers. Drizzle with olive oil and balsamic vinegar.

10. **<u>Egg and Spinach Breakfast Wrap</u>**

Prep Time: 15 minutes

Ingredients: Whole wheat wrap, scrambled eggs, sautéed spinach, cherry tomatoes

Method: Fill a wrap with scrambled eggs, sautéed spinach, and sliced cherry tomatoes. Roll it up and enjoy.

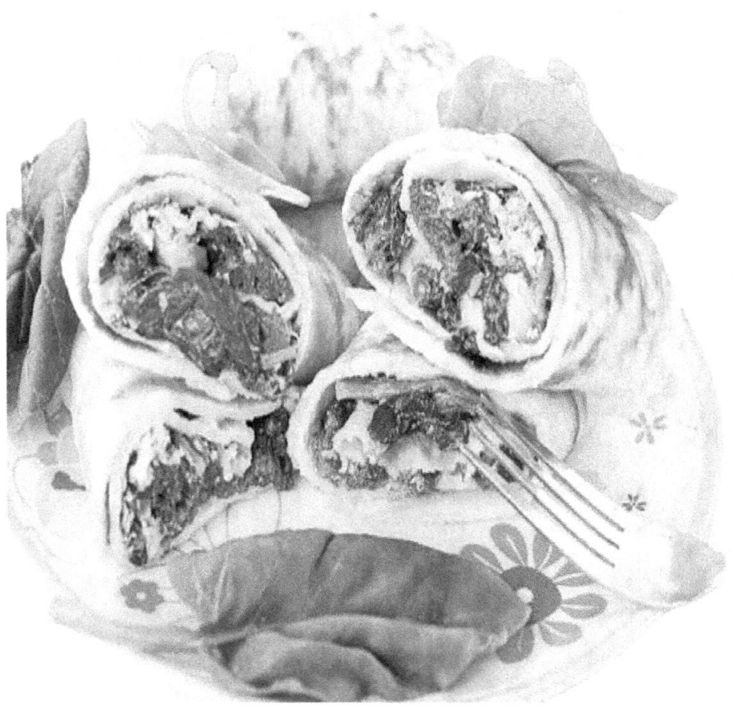

11. **Greek Style Oatmeal**

Prep Time: 10 minutes

Ingredients: Rolled oats, almond milk, honey, cinnamon, chopped nuts

Method:

1. Cook oats with almond milk until creamy.
2. Stir in honey, cinnamon, and chopped nuts and then serve.

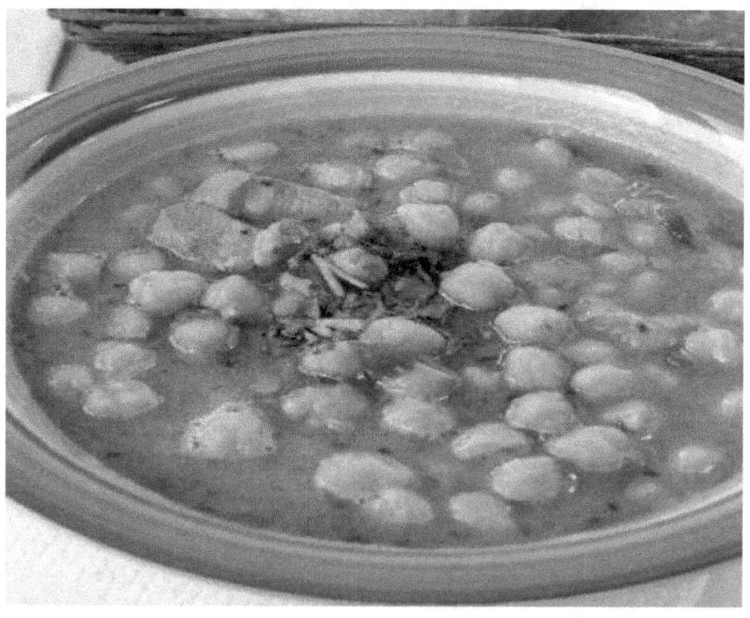

12. **<u>Mediterranean Chia Seed Pudding</u>**

Prep Time: 5 minutes (plus chilling time)

Ingredients: Chia seeds, coconut milk, honey, mixed berries

Method:

1. Mix chia seeds with coconut milk and honey in a jar.
2. Refrigerate overnight.
3. Top with mixed berries before serving it.

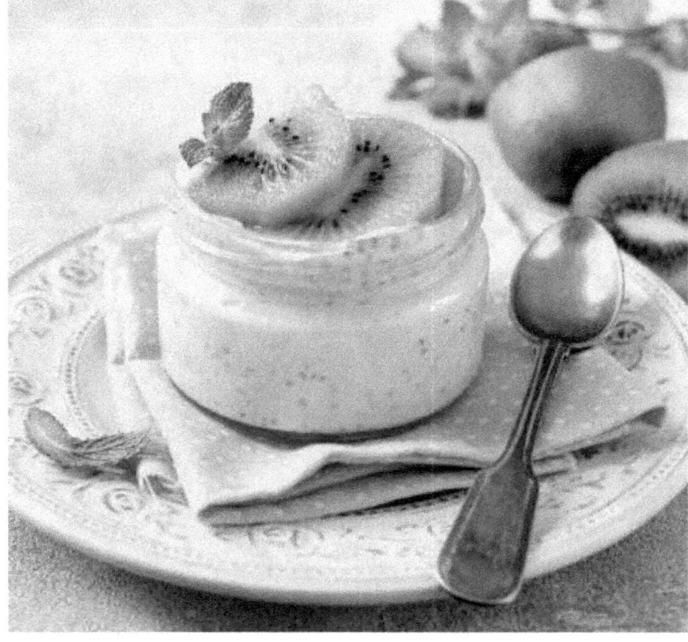

13. **<u>Turkish Menemen</u>**

Prep Time: 25 minutes

Ingredients: Eggs, tomatoes, green peppers, onions, garlic, olive oil

Method:

1. Sauté onions and garlic in olive oil.
2. Add chopped tomatoes and green peppers.
3. Break eggs into the mixture and cook until set.

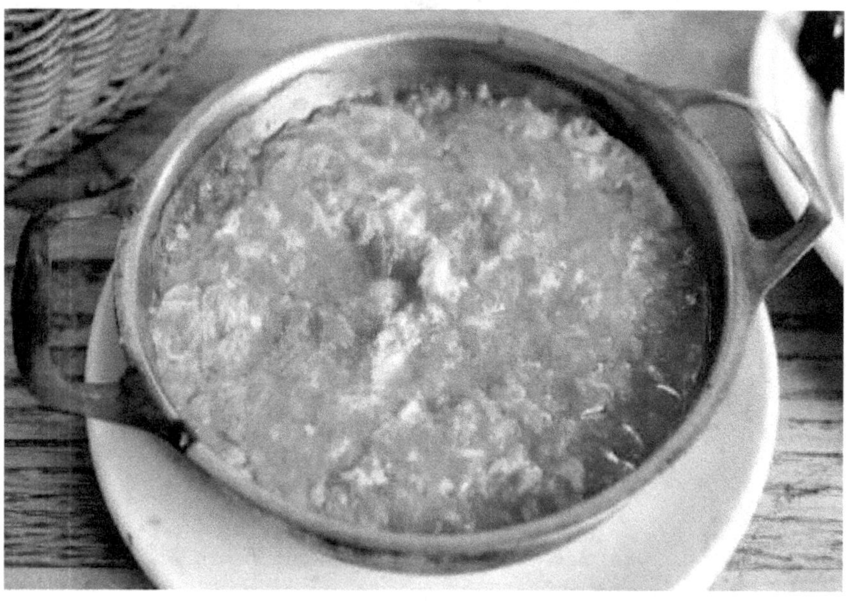

14. <u>**Greek Style Breakfast Bowl**</u>

Prep Time: 15 minutes

Ingredients: Quinoa, Greek yogurt, honey, almonds, figs

Method:

1. Cook quinoa according to package instructions.
2. Top with Greek yogurt, honey-drizzled almonds, and sliced figs.

15. <u>**Mediterranean Breakfast Salad**</u>

Prep Time: 15 minutes

Ingredients: Mixed greens, hard-boiled eggs, chickpeas, cucumbers, feta cheese

Method:

1. Toss mixed greens with chickpeas, sliced hard-boiled eggs, cucumbers, and crumbled feta cheese.
2. Drizzle with olive oil and lemon juice.

16. <u>Spanakopita Muffins</u>

Prep Time: 30 minutes

Ingredients: Spinach, feta cheese, phyllo dough sheets

Method

1. Mix cooked spinach with crumbled feta cheese.
2. Cut phyllo dough sheets into squares and fill each with the spinach mixture.
3. Bake until golden brown.

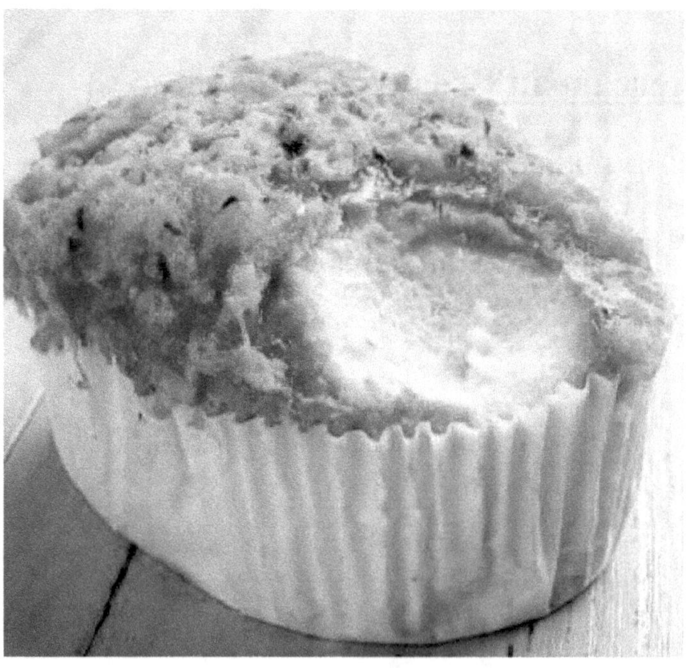

17. <u>Mediterranean Breakfast Bruschetta</u>

Prep Time: 15 minutes

Ingredients: Whole grain baguette slices, hummus, cherry tomatoes, cucumbers

Method:

1. Toast baguette slices and spread hummus on top.
2. Top with diced cherry tomatoes and cucumbers.

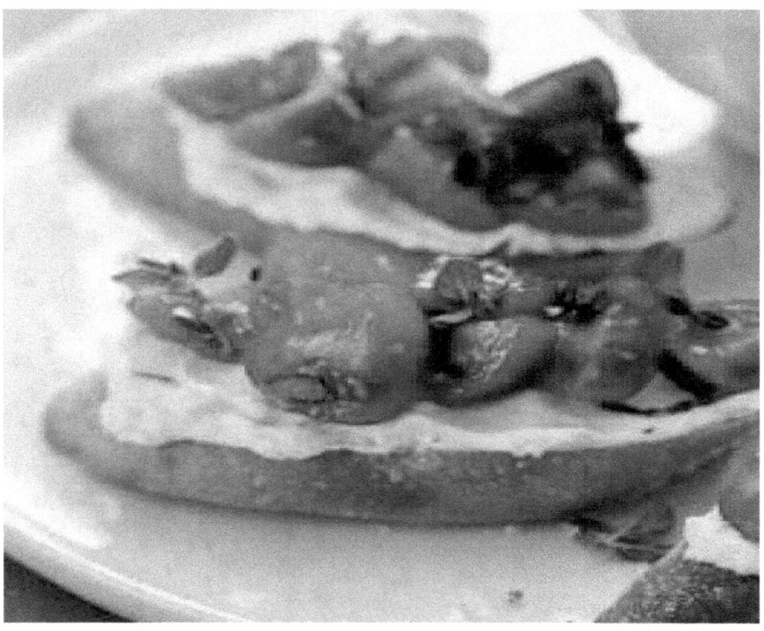

18. <u>Moroccan Style Breakfast Couscous</u>

Prep Time: 20 minutes

Ingredients: Couscous, almond milk, dried fruits (dates/apricots), nuts (almonds/pistachios), cinnamon

Method:

1. Cook couscous in almond milk until fluffy.
2. Stir well in dried fruits and nuts.
3. Sprinkle with cinnamon before serving.

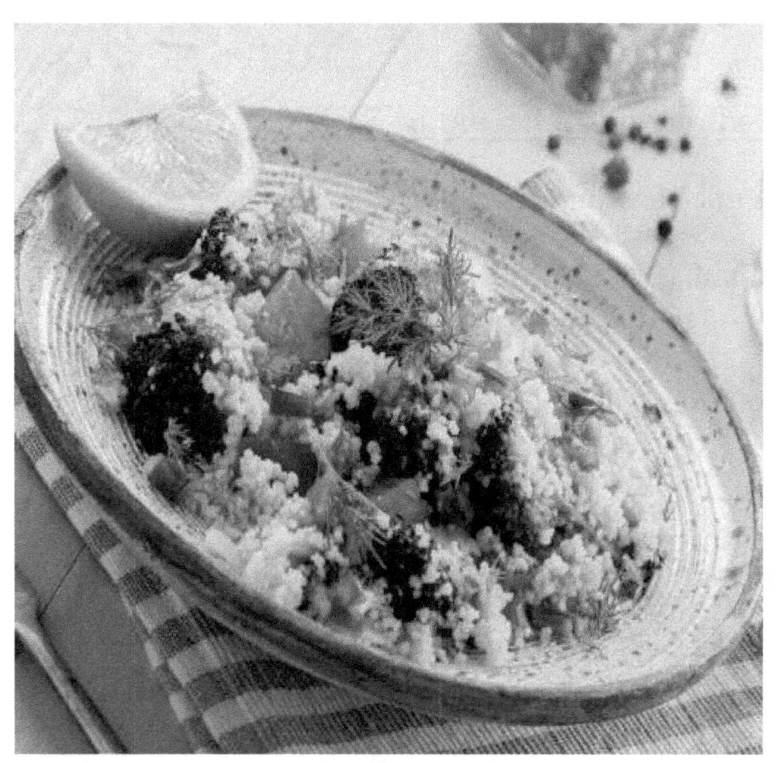

19. <u>Mediterranean Breakfast Smoothie Bowl</u>

Prep Time: 10 minutes

Ingredients: Frozen mixed berries, banana, Greek yogurt, honey, granola

Method:

1. Blend mixed berries with banana and Greek yogurt until smooth.
2. Pour the mixture into a bowl and top with honey and granola.

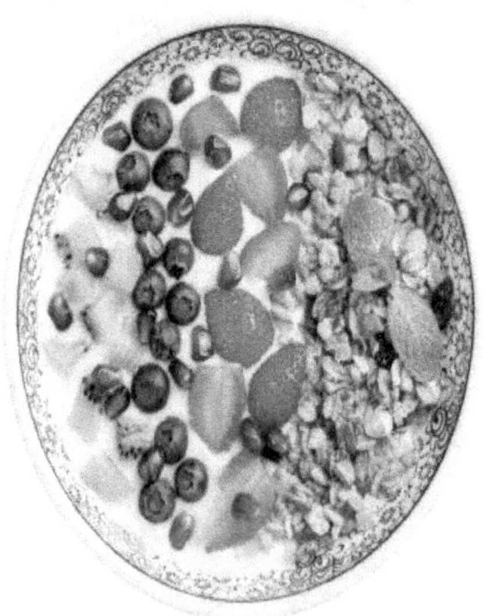

20. <u>Lebanese Labneh Toasts</u>

Prep Time: 10 minutes

Ingredients: Whole grain bread slices, labneh (strained yogurt), za'atar spice blend

Method:

1. Spread labneh on toasted bread slices.
2. Sprinkle with za'atar spice blend it before serving.

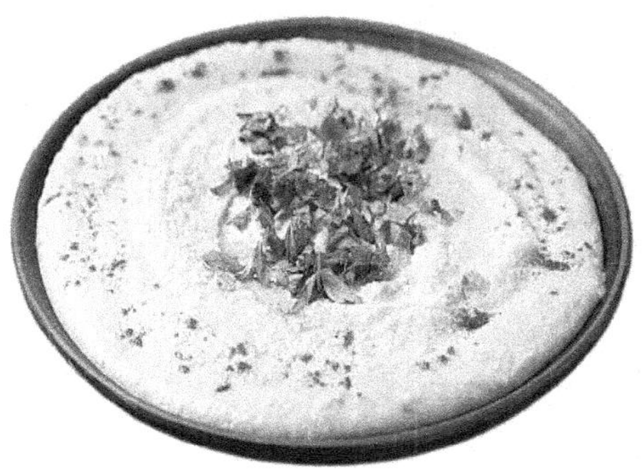

Enjoy these healthful Mediterranean-inspired breakfast dishes as you begin your pregnancy!

CHAPTER FOUR

Energizing Lunch Ideas

1. Mediterranean Chickpea Salad

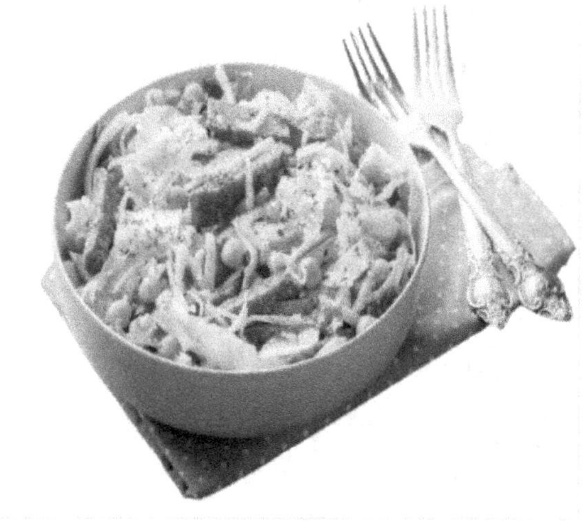

Prep Time: 15 minutes

Ingredients: Chickpeas, cucumbers, cherry tomatoes, red onion, feta cheese, olives, lemon juice, olive oil

Method:

1. Combine all ingredients in a bowl and toss with lemon juice and olive oil.

2.Spread with crumbled feta cheese.

2. <u>Greek Quinoa Salad</u>

Prep Time: 20 minutes

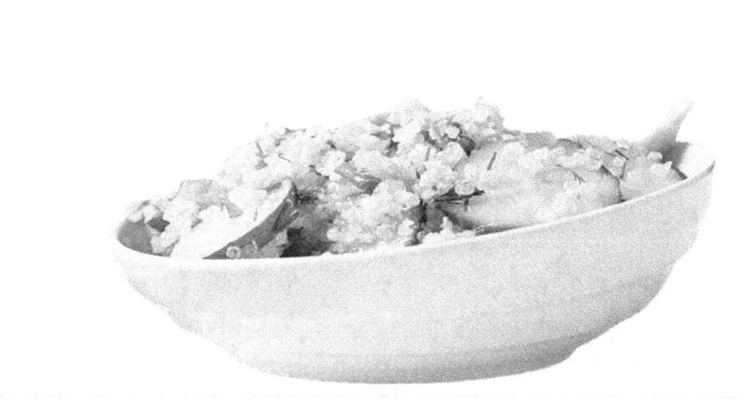

Ingredients: Quinoa, bell peppers, cucumbers, red onion, Kalamata olives, feta cheese, lemon vinaigrette

Method:

1.Cook quinoa according to package instructions.
2.Mix in chopped vegetables, olives, and feta cheese.
3.Drizzle with lemon vinaigrette and enjoy.

3. <u>Falafel Wrap</u>

Prep Time: 30 minutes

Ingredients: Falafel balls, whole wheat wrap, hummus, tzatziki sauce, lettuce, tomatoes, cucumbers

Method:

1. Heat falafel balls according to package instructions.
2. Fill a wrap with falafel, hummus, tzatziki sauce, and fresh vegetables.
3. Roll up and enjoy!

4. <u>Mediterranean Stuffed Bell Peppers</u>

Prep Time: 40 minutes

Ingredients: Bell peppers, quinoa, chickpeas, tomatoes, feta cheese, olives, herbs

Method:

1. Cut the tops off bell peppers and remove seeds.
2. Stuff with a mixture of cooked quinoa, chickpeas, diced tomatoes, feta cheese, olives, and herbs.
3. Bake until peppers are tender, Enjoy.

5. <u>Greek Chicken Pita Pockets</u>

Prep Time: 25 minutes

Ingredients: Grilled chicken strips, whole wheat pita bread, Greek yogurt, cucumber, tomatoes, red onion

Method:

Fill pita pockets with grilled chicken strips, Greek yogurt, diced cucumbers, tomatoes, and red onion, enjoy.

6. <u>Lemon Herb Salmon Salad</u>

Prep Time: 20 minutes

Ingredients: Grilled salmon fillet, mixed greens, cherry tomatoes, avocado, lemon herb dressing

Method:

1. Flake grilled salmon over a bed of mixed greens.
2. Add cherry tomatoes and sliced avocado.
3. Drizzle with lemon herb dressing.

7. <u>Mediterranean Veggie Wrap</u>

Prep Time: 15 minutes

Ingredients: Roasted vegetables (zucchini, bell peppers, eggplant), hummus, feta cheese, spinach leaves

Method:

1.Spread hummus on a whole wheat wrap.
2.Add roasted vegetables, crumbled feta cheese, and spinach leaves.
3.Roll up and enjoy!

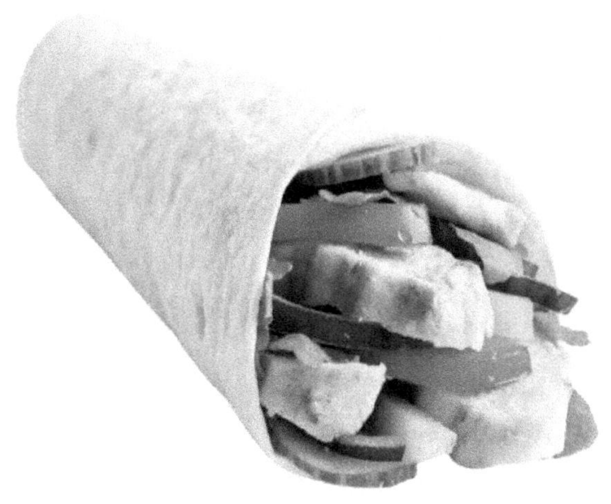

8. <u>Greek Lentil Soup</u>

Prep Time: 30 minutes

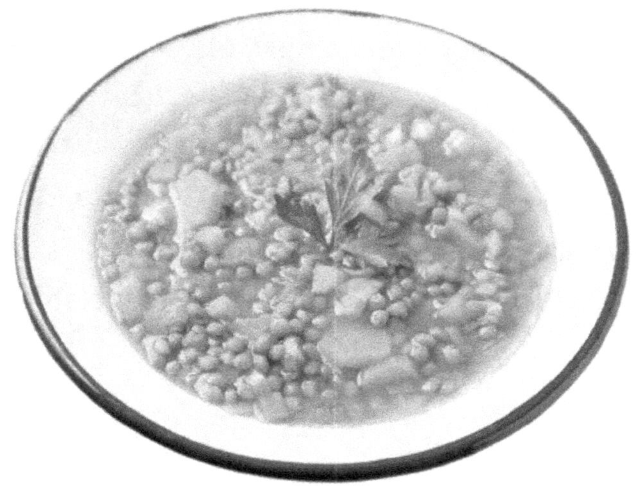

Ingredients: Lentils, carrots, celery, onions, garlic, tomatoes, spinach, lemon juice

Method:

1. Sauté onions, carrots, celery, and garlic in a pot.
2. Add lentils, diced tomatoes, and vegetable broth.
3. Simmer until lentils are tender. Stir in spinach and lemon juice before serving.

9. <u>Mediterranean Quinoa Bowl</u>

Prep Time: 25 minutes

Ingredients: Quinoa, grilled chicken strips, roasted vegetables (bell peppers, zucchini), olives, feta cheese

Method:

1. Cook quinoa according to package instructions.
2. Spread with grilled chicken strips, roasted vegetables, olives, and crumbled feta cheese.

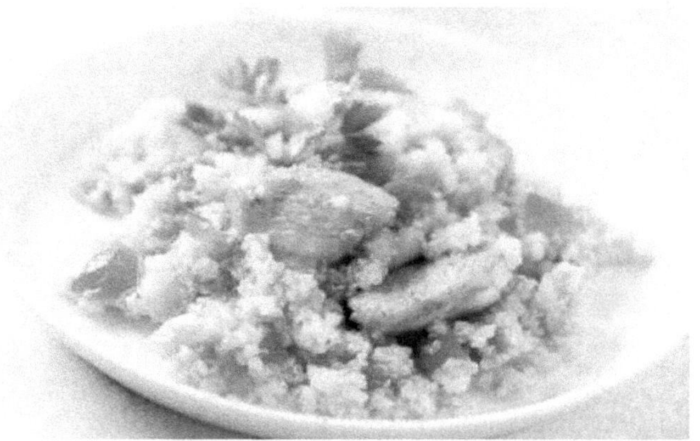

10. <u>Greek Orzo Salad</u>

Prep Time: 20 minutes

Ingredients: Orzo pasta, cherry tomatoes, cucumbers, red onion, feta cheese, olives, lemon vinaigrette

Method:

1. Cook orzo pasta according to package instructions.
2. Mix in chopped vegetables, feta cheese, olives, and drizzle with lemon vinaigrette.

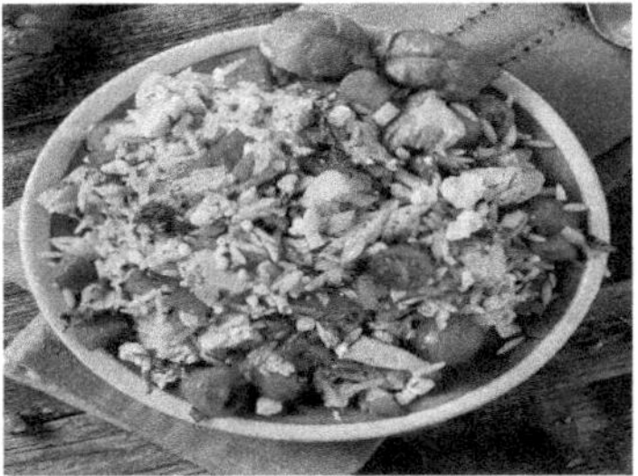

11. <u>Mediterranean Hummus Plate</u>

Prep Time: 15 minutes

Ingredients: Hummus, falafel balls, grape leaves, tabbouleh salad, pita bread

Method:

Arrange hummus in a plate and surround it with falafel balls, grape leaves, tabbouleh salad, and pita bread for dipping.

12. <u>Greek Chicken Salad Bowl</u>

Prep Time: 25 minutes

Ingredients: Grilled chicken breast slices, mixed greens, cherry tomatoes, cucumbers, feta cheese

Method:

1. Arrange mixed greens in a bowl.
2. Top with grilled chicken breast slices, cherry tomatoes, cucumbers, and crumbled feta cheese.

13. <u>Mediterranean Tuna Salad Wraps</u>

Prep Time: 20 minutes

Ingredients: Canned tuna in olive oil, mixed greens, cherry tomatoes, red onion, olives, whole wheat wraps

Method:

1. Mix canned tuna with chopped vegetables.
2. Fill wraps with tuna salad and mixed greens.
3. Roll up and enjoy.

14. <u>Lemon Garlic Shrimp Pasta</u>

Prep Time: 30 minutes

Ingredients: Shrimp, whole wheat pasta, cherry tomatoes, spinach, garlic, lemon zest

Method:

1. Cook whole wheat pasta according to package instructions.
2. Sauté shrimp with garlic until cooked.
3. Toss pasta with shrimp mixture and add cherry tomatoes, spinach, and lemon zest.

15. <u>Mediterranean Mezze Platter</u>

Prep Time: 20 minutes

Ingredients: Hummus, tzatziki sauce, stuffed grape leaves, olives, pita bread triangles

Method:

1. Arrange hummus and tzatziki sauce in a platter.
2. Add stuffed grape leaves and olives.
3. Serve with pita bread triangles for dipping.

16. <u>Greek Turkey Burgers</u>

Prep Time: 30 minutes

Ingredients: Ground turkey meat, feta cheese crumbles, spinach leaves, red onion slices

Method:

1. Mix ground turkey meat with feta cheese crumbles.
2. Form into patties and grill until cooked through.
3. Serve on whole wheat buns with spinach leaves and red onion slices.

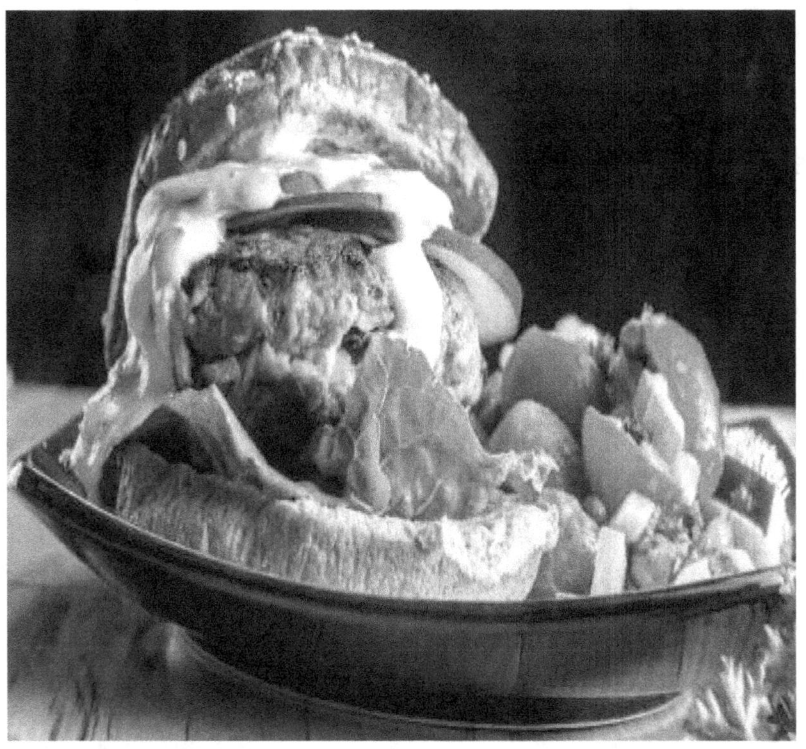

17. <u>Mediterranean Chickpea Stew</u>

Prep Time: 40 minutes

Ingredients: Chickpeas, eggplant, tomatoes, onions, garlic, cumin, coriander

Method:

1. Sauté onions and garlic in a pot.
2. Add diced eggplant and cook until softened.
3. Stir in chickpeas and diced tomatoes.
4. Season with cumin and coriander.

5.Simmer until flavors meld together.

18. <u>Greek Spinach Pie (Spanakopita)</u>

Prep Time: 45 minutes

Ingredients: Phyllo dough sheets, spinach, feta cheese, dill

Method:

1.Layer phyllo dough sheets with a mixture of cooked spinach and crumbled feta cheese seasoned with dill.
2.Bake until golden brown.

19. <u>Mediterranean Quinoa Stuffed Peppers</u>

Prep Time: 45 minutes

Ingredients: Bell peppers, quinoa, black beans, corn kernels, diced tomatoes

Method:

1.Cut the tops off bell peppers and remove seeds.
2.Fill with a mixture of cooked quinoa mixed with black beans, corn kernels and diced tomatoes.
3.Bake until peppers are tender and enjoy.

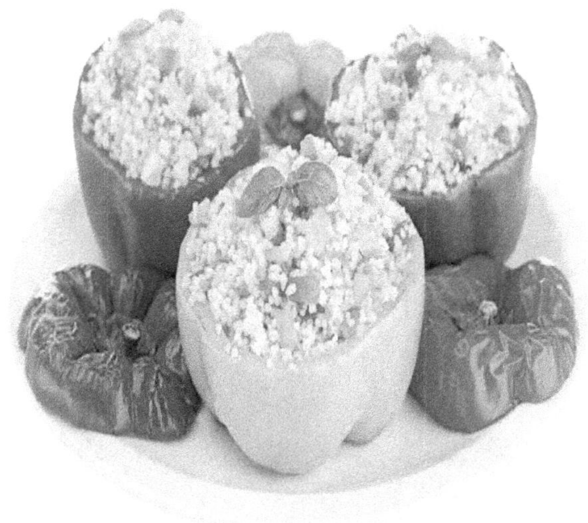

20. <u>Greek Lemon Chicken Soup (Avgolemono)</u>

Prep Time: 30 minutes

Ingredients: Chicken broth/stock (homemade or store-bought), cooked shredded chicken breast meat or rotisserie chicken meat), eggs (beaten), lemon juice.

Method:

1. Put the cooked, shredded chicken flesh into a saucepan with boiling chicken broth or stock, then whisk in the lemon juice and beaten eggs.

2. To temper the egg mixture, gently whisk in a little amount of hot stock.

3. Then, slowly whisk the tempered egg mixture back into the saucepan of hot broth, stirring continuously until the soup slightly thickens.

4. Season with salt and pepper to taste.

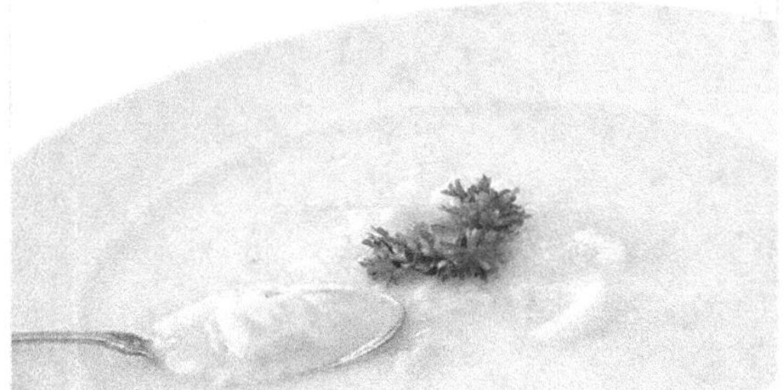

CHAPTER FIVE

Satisfying Dinner Options

1. <u>Mediterranean Stuffed Bell Peppers</u>

Prep Time: 45 minutes

Ingredients:

- 4 bell peppers, halved and seeds removed

- 1 cup cooked quinoa

- 1 can (14 oz) chickpeas, drained and rinsed

- 1/2 cup diced tomatoes

- 1/4 cup chopped Kalamata olives

- 1/4 cup crumbled feta cheese

- 1 teaspoon dried oregano

- Salt and pepper to taste

Method:

1. Preheat the oven to 375°F.

2. In a large bowl, mix together the cooked quinoa, chickpeas, diced tomatoes, olives, feta cheese, oregano, salt, and pepper.

3. Stuff the bell pepper halves with the quinoa mixture.

4. Place the stuffed peppers in a baking dish and cover with foil.

5. Bake for 30 minutes, then remove the foil and bake for an additional 10 minutes until the peppers are tender.

6. Serve hot and enjoy this nutritious and satisfying meal.

2. <u>Mediterranean Chickpea Salad</u>

Prep Time: 20 minutes

Ingredients:

- 1 can (14 oz) chickpeas, drained and rinsed

- 1 cucumber, diced

- 1 bell pepper, diced

- 1/2 red onion, thinly sliced

- 1/4 cup chopped fresh parsley

- Juice of 1 lemon

- 2 tablespoons olive oil

- Salt and pepper to taste

Method:

1. In a large bowl, combine the chickpeas, cucumber, bell pepper, red onion, and parsley.

2. In a small bowl, whisk together the lemon juice, olive oil, salt, and pepper.

3. Pour the dressing over the salad and toss to combine.

4. Chill in the refrigerator for at least 30 minutes before serving.

5. Enjoy this refreshing and protein-packed Mediterranean Chickpea Salad.

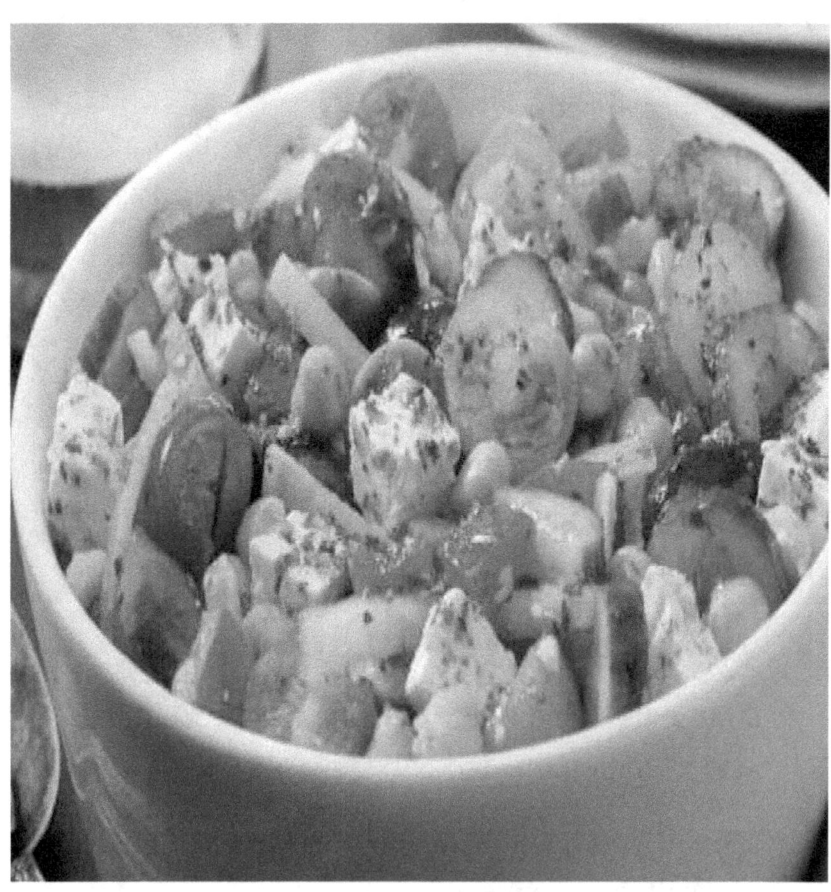

3. <u>Mediterranean Lentil Tabbouleh</u>

Prep Time: 30 minutes

Ingredients:

- 1 cup cooked green lentils

- 1 cup cooked bulgur wheat

- 1 cucumber, diced

- 1 tomato, diced

- 1/4 cup chopped fresh mint

- 1/4 cup chopped fresh parsley

- Juice of 1 lemon

- 2 tablespoons olive oil

- Salt and pepper to taste

Method:

1. In a large bowl, combine the cooked lentils, bulgur wheat, cucumber, tomato, mint, and parsley.

2. In a small bowl, whisk together the lemon juice, olive oil, salt, and pepper.

3. Pour the dressing over the tabbouleh and toss to combine.

4. Chill in the refrigerator for at least 20 minutes before serving.

5. Enjoy this flavorful and nutrient-rich

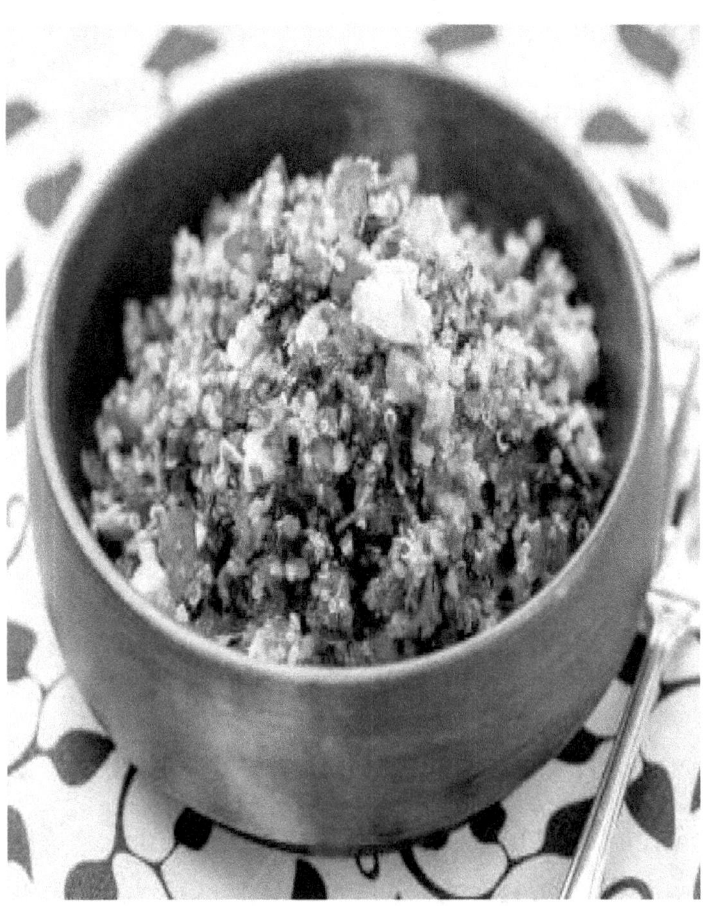

4. <u>Mediterranean Roasted Vegetable Platter</u>

Prep Time: 40 minutes

Ingredients:

- 1 eggplant, sliced into rounds

- 1 zucchini, sliced into rounds

- 1 red bell pepper, sliced into strips

- 1 yellow bell pepper, sliced into strips

- 1 red onion, sliced into wedges

- 2 tablespoons olive oil

- 1 teaspoon dried thyme

- Salt and pepper to taste

Method:

1. Preheat the oven to 400°F.

2. Place the sliced vegetables on a baking sheet.

3. Drizzle with olive oil and sprinkle with thyme, salt, and pepper.

4. Roast in the oven for 30-35 minutes, or until the vegetables are tender and slightly caramelized.

5. Arrange the roasted vegetables on a platter and serve as a colorful and delicious Mediterranean-inspired meal.

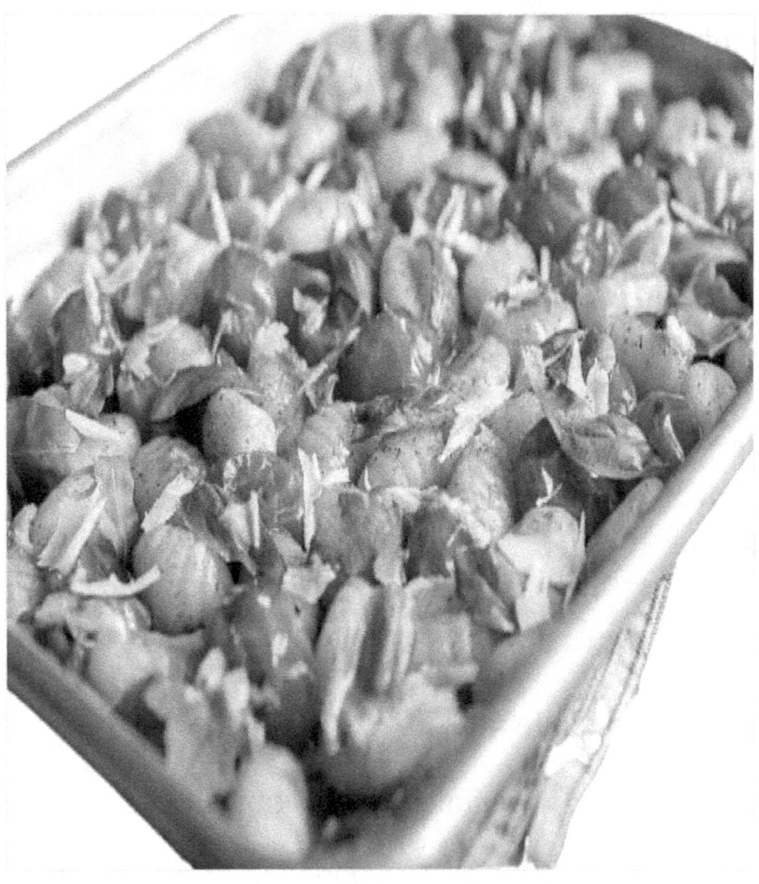

5. <u>Mediterranean Quinoa Bowl with Lemon Tahini Dressing</u>

Prep Time: 30 minutes

Ingredients:

- 1 cup cooked quinoa

- 1 can (14 oz) chickpeas, drained and rinsed

- 1 cucumber, diced

- 1 tomato, diced

- 1/4 cup crumbled feta cheese

- Juice of 1 lemon

- 2 tablespoons tahini

- 2 tablespoons water

- Salt and pepper to taste

Method:

1. In a bowl, combine the cooked quinoa, chickpeas, cucumber, tomato, and feta cheese.

2. In a small bowl, whisk together the lemon juice, tahini, water, salt, and pepper to make the dressing.

3. Pour the dressing over the quinoa bowl and toss to combine.

4. Serve this nutritious and flavorful Mediterranean Quinoa Bowl for a satisfying dinner option.

6. <u>Mediterranean Baked Falafel with Tzatziki Sauce</u>

Prep Time: 45 minutes

Ingredients:

For the falafel:

- 1 can (14 oz) chickpeas, drained and rinsed

- 2 cloves garlic, minced

- 1/4 cup chopped fresh parsley

- 1 teaspoon ground cumin

- 1/2 teaspoon ground coriander

- Salt and pepper to taste

For the tzatziki sauce:

- 1 cup Greek yogurt

- 1/2 cucumber, grated and excess water squeezed out

- 2 cloves garlic, minced

- Juice of 1 lemon

- Salt and pepper to taste

Method:

For the falafel:

1. Preheat the oven to 375°F.

2. In a food processor, pulse the

chickpeas, garlic, parsley, cumin, coriander, salt, and pepper until combined but still slightly chunky.

3. Form the mixture into small patties and place on a baking sheet lined with parchment paper.

4. Bake for 25-30 minutes until golden brown and crispy.

For the tzatziki sauce:

5. In a bowl, mix together the Greek yogurt, grated cucumber, garlic, lemon juice, salt, and pepper.

6. Serve the baked falafel with tzatziki sauce for a delicious Mediterranean-inspired dinner.

7. <u>Mediterranean Lemon Herb Chicken Skewers with Tzatziki Sauce</u>

Prep Time: 40 minutes

Ingredients:

For the chicken skewers:

- 1 lb chicken breast or thigh meat, cut into cubes

- Zest of 1 lemon

- Juice of 1 lemon

- 2 cloves garlic, minced

- 2 tablespoons chopped fresh parsley

- 2 tablespoons chopped fresh oregano

- Salt and pepper to taste

For the tzatziki sauce:

- 1 cup Greek yogurt

- 1/2 cucumber, grated and excess water squeezed out

- 2 cloves garlic, minced

- Juice of 1 lemon

- Salt and pepper to taste

Method:

For the chicken skewers:

1. In a bowl, combine the chicken cubes with lemon zest, lemon juice, garlic, parsley, oregano, salt, and pepper.

2. Thread the marinated chicken onto skewers.

3. Grill or bake the skewers until cooked through.

For the tzatziki sauce:

4. In a bowl, mix together the Greek yogurt, grated cucumber, garlic, lemon juice, salt, and pepper.

5. Serve the Mediterranean Lemon Herb Chicken Skewers with Tzatziki Sauce for a flavorful and satisfying dinner option.

8. <u>Mediterranean Baked Eggplant Parmesan</u>

Prep Time: 50 minutes

Ingredients:

- 2 eggplants, sliced into rounds

- Salt for sweating eggplant slices

For the tomato sauce:

- 1 can (14 oz) diced tomatoes

- 2 cloves garlic, minced

- 1 teaspoon dried oregano

- Salt and pepper to taste

For assembly:

- Olive oil for brushing eggplant slices

- Mozzarella cheese slices or shredded cheese of choice (optional)

Method:

1. Preheat the oven to 375°F.

2. Place eggplant slices on a baking sheet and sprinkle with salt to draw out moisture.

3. After about 15 minutes, pat dry the eggplant slices with paper towels.

4. Brush both sides of eggplant slices with olive oil and bake for about 20 minutes until tender.

5. In a saucepan, combine diced tomatoes with garlic, oregano, salt, and pepper. Simmer for about 10 minutes to make tomato sauce.

6. Layer baked eggplant slices in a baking dish with tomato sauce and optional cheese between layers.

7. Bake for an additional 15 minutes until cheese is melted and bubbly.

8. Serve hot as a comforting Mediterranean Baked Eggplant Parmesan.

9. <u>Mediterranean Lemon Garlic Shrimp Pasta</u>

Prep Time: 30 minutes

Ingredients:

- 8 oz pasta of choice

- 1 lb shrimp

- Zest of one lemon

- Juice of one lemon

- 3 cloves garlic

- Olive oil

- Fresh parsley

- Salt & pepper

Method:

Cook pasta according to package instructions.

In a skillet over medium heat cook shrimp in olive oil until pink on both sides (about three minutes per side). Add minced garlic halfway through cooking shrimp.

Add lemon zest & juice to shrimp in skillet; mix well
to coat shrimp.

Once pasta is done cooking drain & add to skillet
with shrimp; toss well to combine ingredients.

Serve hot garnished with fresh parsley.

10. <u>Mediterranean Grilled Vegetable Platter</u>

Prep Time: 30 minutes

Ingredients:

-Zucchini

-Eggplant

-Bell peppers

-Onions

-Olive oil

-Garlic powder

-Dried oregano

-Salt & pepper

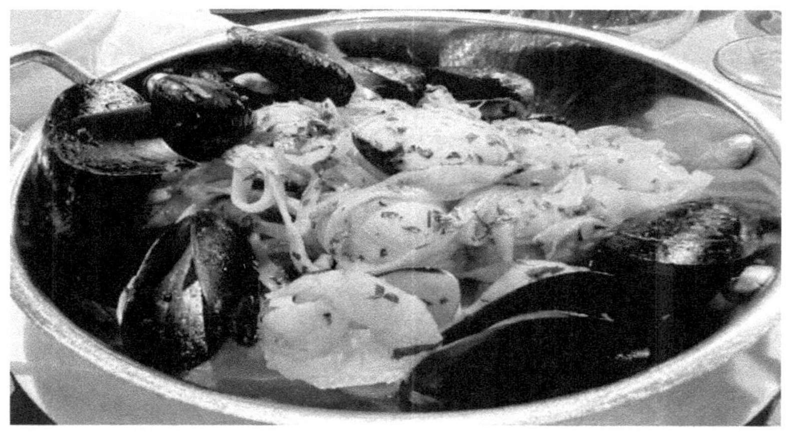

Method:

1. Slice vegetables into even pieces & brush with olive oil;
2. Season with garlic powder & dried oregano; sprinkle with salt & pepper
3. Grill vegetables over medium heat until tender & grill marks appear (about five minutes per side).

   Arrange grilled vegetables on platter & serve hot as a colorful & flavorful meal.

11. <u>Mediterranean Chickpea Stew with Spinach</u>

Prep Time: One hour

Ingredients:

-Chickpeas

-Onion

-Garlic

-Carrots

-Celery

-Tomato paste

-Vegetable broth

-Spinach

-Cumin

-Coriander

-Smoked paprika

-Salt & pepper

Method:

1. In a large pot cook onion & garlic until softened; add carrots & celery & cook until tender (about five minutes).
2. Add chickpeas & tomato paste; stir well to coat chickpeas in paste.
3. Pour in vegetable broth & season with cumin; coriander; smoked paprika; salt & pepper; bring to boil then reduce heat & simmer for thirty minutes until chickpeas are tender & flavors are melded together;
4. Add spinach & cook until wilted (about five minutes).
5. Serve hot as a hearty & nutritious stew.

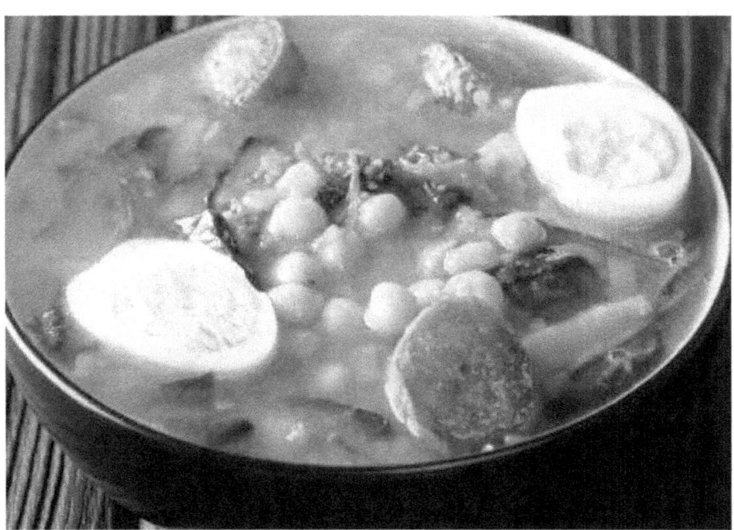

12. <u>Mediterranean Quinoa Salad with Roasted Vegetables</u>

Prep Time: One hour

Ingredients:

Quinoa

Zucchini

Red bell peppers

Cherry tomatoes

Red onion

Olive oil

Lemon juice

Garlic powder

Dried oregano

Salt & pepper

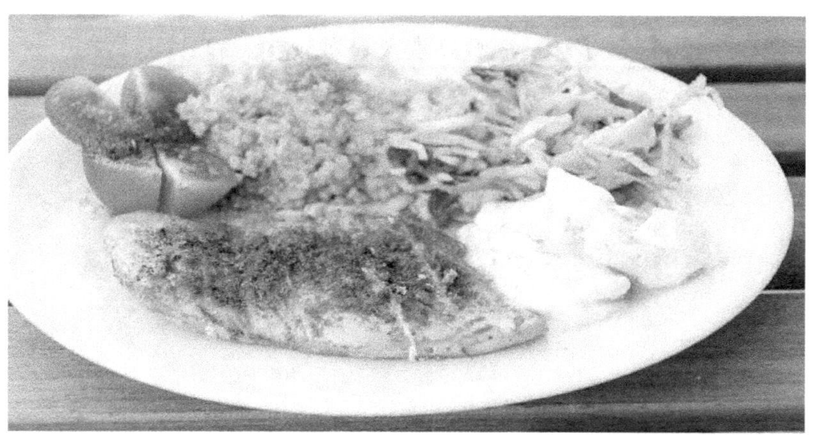

Method:

1. Cook quinoa according to package instructions; set aside to cool
2. Toss zucchini; red bell peppers; cherry tomatoes; red onion in olive oil; season with garlic powder; dried oregano; salt & pepper
3. Roast vegetables in oven at four hundred degrees Fahrenheit until tender (about thirty minutes); let cool
4. In large bowl combine cooked quinoa & roasted vegetables; drizzle with olive oil & lemon juice; toss well to combine
5. Serve chilled as a refreshing & nutrient-packed salad

13. <u>**Mediterranean Lentil Soup with Spinach**</u>

Prep Time: Forty-five minutes

Ingredients:

Green or brown lentils

Onion

Garlic

Carrot

Celery

Diced tomatoes

Vegetable broth

Cumin

Coriander

Smoked paprika

Salt & pepper

Spinach

Lemon juice

Fresh parsley or cilantro

Method:

Heat olive oil in pot over medium heat; add onion; garlic; carrot; celery; cook until softened (about five minutes). Add lentils; diced tomatoes; vegetable broth; cumin; coriander; smoked paprika; salt & pepper; stir well to combine; bring soup to boil then reduce heat & simmer for thirty-five minutes until lentils are tender

Stir in spinach & lemon juice; cook an additional five minutes until spinach is wilted

Taste & adjust seasoning if needed

Ladle soup into bowls & garnish with fresh parsley or cilantro if desired

Serve hot as a comforting & nutritious meal

14. <u>Mediterranean Grilled Chicken Skewers with Greek Salad</u>

Prep Time: One hour

Ingredients:

Chicken breast

Lemon zest

Lemon juice

Garlic

Olive oil

Greek yogurt

Cucumber

Garlic

Lemon juice

Salt & pepper

Cucumber

Tomato

Red onion

Kalamata olives

Feta cheese

Olive oil

Red wine vinegar

Dried oregano

Salt & pepper

Method:

Marinate chicken breast in mixture of lemon zest; lemon juice; minced garlic; olive oil; Greek yogurt; salt & pepper for thirty minutes

Thread marinated chicken onto skewers

Grill chicken skewers over medium heat until cooked through (about ten minutes per side)

Prepare Greek salad by combining diced cucumber; tomato; red onion; Kalamata olives; crumbled feta cheese in large bowl

In small bowl whisk together olive oil; red wine vinegar; dried oregano; salt & pepper pour dressing over salad toss well to combine

Serve grilled chicken skewers with Greek salad for a delicious & satisfying meal

15. <u>Mediterranean Baked Salmon with Lemon Herb Butter</u>

Prep Time: Thirty-five minutes

Ingredients:

Salmon fillets

Butter

Lemon zest

Lemon juice

Garlic

Fresh parsley

Fresh dill

Salt & pepper

Method:

1.Preheat oven to four hundred degrees Fahrenheit

2.In small saucepan melt butter over low heat;
3.Stir in lemon zest; lemon juice; minced garlic; chopped
    parsley; chopped dill; salt & pepper
4.Place salmon fillets on baking sheet lined with
    parchment paper; spoon lemon herb butter over
    salmon fillets
5.Bake salmon in oven for fifteen-twenty minutes until
    salmon is cooked through
6.Serve hot as a flavorful & healthy dinner option

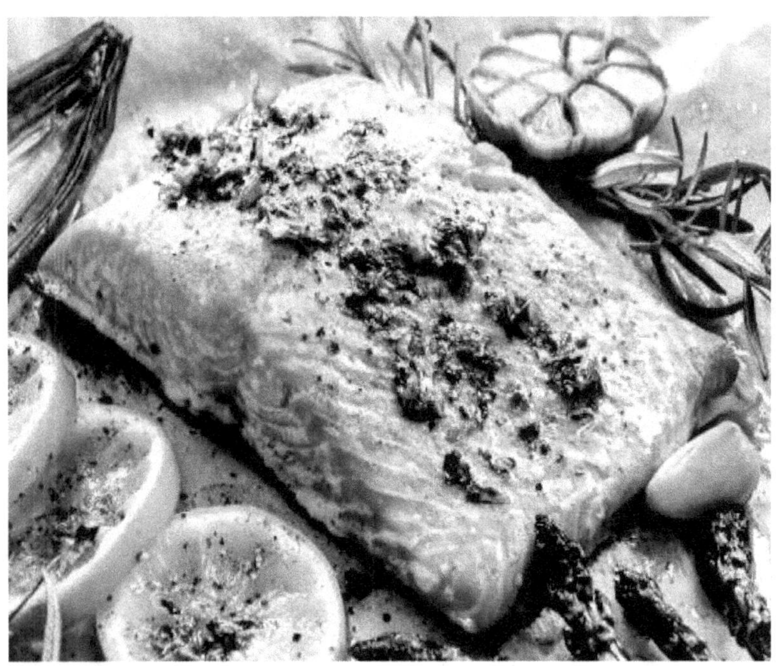

16. <u>Mediterranean Baked Falafel Bowl</u>

Prep Time: One hour

Ingredients:

- Chickpeas
- Garlic
- Fresh parsley
- Ground cumin
- Ground coriander
- Salt & pepper
- Greek yogurt
- Cucumber
- Garlic
- Lemon juice
- Salt & pepper
- Cooked quinoa or rice
- Cherry tomatoes
- Cucumber
- Red onion
- Kalamata olives

- Feta cheese
- Olive oil
- Lemon juice
- Dried oregano
- Salt & pepper

Method:

In food processor pulse chickpeas; garlic; parsley; cumin; coriander; salt & pepper until combined but still slightly chunky form mixture into small patties place on baking sheet lined with parchment paper bake for twenty-five-thirty minutes until golden brown & crispy prepare tzatziki sauce by mixing together Greek yogurt; grated cucumber; garlic; lemon juice; salt & pepper in bowl cook quinoa or rice according to package instructions divide cooked quinoa or rice among bowls top with baked falafel patties cherry tomatoes cucumber red onion Kalamata olives feta cheese drizzle bowls with olive oil lemon juice sprinkle with dried oregano salt & pepper serve hot as a satisfying Mediterranean-inspired meal option.

17. <u>Mediterranean Lemon Herb Roasted Chicken Thighs</u>

Prep Time: Forty-five minutes

Ingredients:

Chicken thighs

Lemon zest

Lemon juice

Garlic

Fresh parsley

Fresh oregano

Fresh thyme

Olive oil

Salt & pepper

Method:

Preheat oven to four hundred degrees Fahrenheit line baking sheet with parchment paper place chicken thighs on baking sheet sprinkle with lemon zest lemon juice minced garlic chopped parsley chopped oregano chopped thyme drizzle with olive oil season with salt & pepper roast chicken thighs in oven for thirty-forty minutes until golden brown & cooked through serve hot as a flavorful & comforting dinner option.

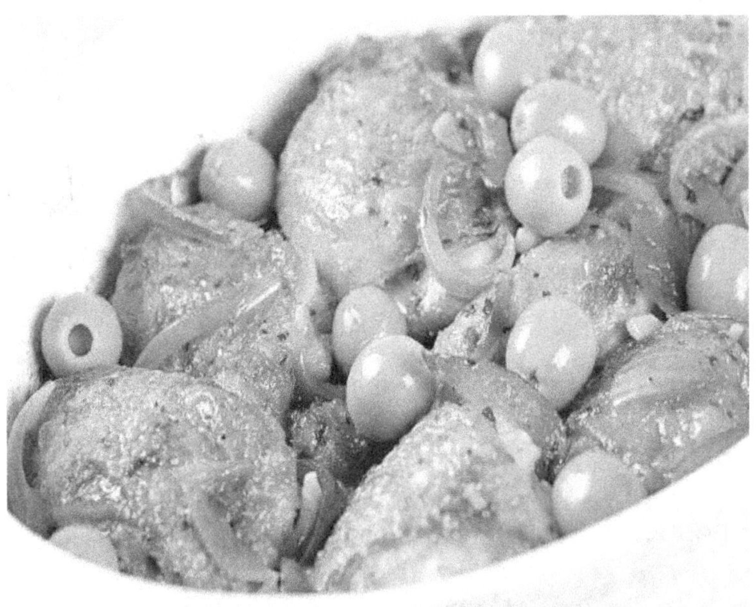

18. <u>Mediterranean Vegetable Frittata</u>

Prep Time: Forty-five minutes

Ingredients:

Eggs

Milk or cream

Red bell pepper

Zucchini

Red onion

Cherry tomatoes

Feta cheese

Fresh parsley or basil

Olive oil

Salt & pepper

Method:

Preheat oven to three hundred fifty degrees
Fahrenheit whisk together eggs milk or cream in bowl
set aside sauté red bell pepper zucchini red onion
cherry tomatoes in oven-safe skillet over medium
heat until vegetables are tender pour egg mixture over
sautéed vegetables crumble feta cheese over top
sprinkle with chopped parsley or basil season with
salt & pepper cook on stovetop for five minutes
transfer skillet to oven bake frittata for twenty-
twenty-five minutes until set serve hot as a nutritious
& satisfying meal.

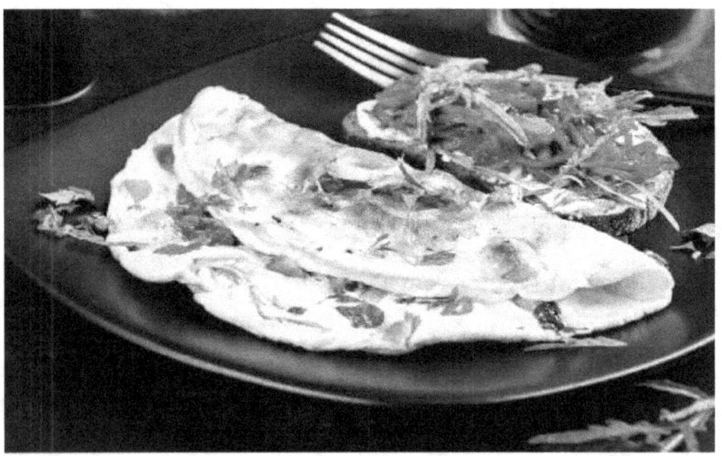

19. <u>Mediterranean Shrimp Scampi Pasta</u>

Prep Time: Thirty-five minutes

Ingredients:

Pasta of choice

Shrimp

Butter

Olive oil

Garlic

Red chili flakes

White wine (optional)

Lemon zest

Lemon juice

Fresh parsley

Salt & pepper

Method:

Cook pasta according to package instructions drain set aside cook shrimp in skillet over medium heat in butter olive oil minced garlic red chili flakes until pink on both sides about three minutes per side add white wine if using halfway through cooking shrimp add lemon zest lemon juice fresh parsley season with salt & pepper once pasta is done cooking drain add to skillet with shrimp toss well to combine ingredients serve hot garnished with fresh parsley as a flavorful dinner option.

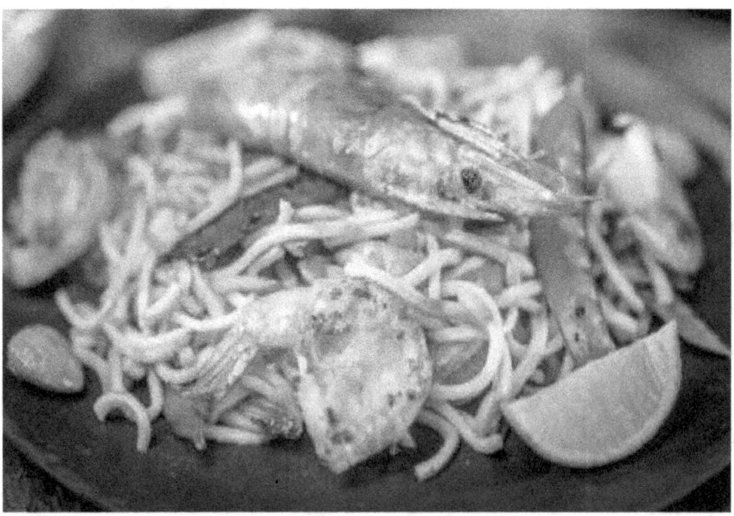

20. <u>Mediterranean Stuffed Portobello Mushrooms</u>

Prep Time: Forty-five minutes

Ingredients:

Portobello mushrooms Olive oil,

Garlic Spinach

Red bell pepper

Cherry tomatoes

Feta cheese

Fresh parsley

Salt & pepper

Method: Preheat oven to four hundred degrees Fahrenheit remove stems from portobello mushrooms brush mushroom caps with olive oil season with minced garlic salt & pepper bake mushrooms in oven for fifteen-twenty minutes until tender meanwhile sauté spinach red bell pepper cherry tomatoes in skillet over medium heat until vegetables are tender fill baked portobello mushrooms with sautéed vegetable mixture crumble feta cheese over top sprinkle with chopped parsley return stuffed mushrooms to oven bake an additional five minutes until cheese is melted serve hot as a flavorful vegetarian dinner option.

These recipes offer a variety of delicious options that are both nourishing and satisfying for expecting moms following a Mediterranean diet plan

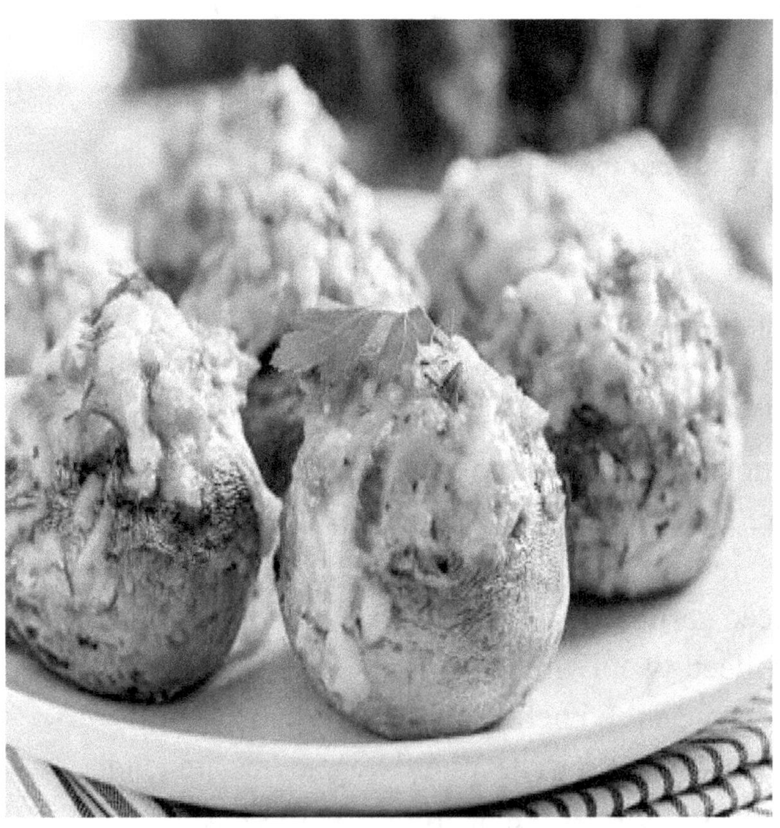

CHAPTER SIX

Snacks and Treats for Pregnancy Cravings

Throughout pregnancy, cravings may strike at any moment, so it's important to have healthy snack options on hand to satisfy your body and your cravings. This chapter will discuss a variety of delicious, high-nutrient snacks and treats that are perfect for expecting moms and go well with a Mediterranean diet. These recipes, which include anything from sweet treats like almond butter banana nibbles and dark chocolate avocado mousse to savory hummus, will let you indulge without jeopardizing the health of your unborn child.

1. <u>Hummus with roasted red pepper and vegetable sticks</u>

20 minutes for preparation

Ingredients:

- One 14-oz can of washed and drained chickpeas
- Half a cup of roasted peppers
- Two garlic cloves
- Two teaspoons of tahini
- One lemon's juice
- Two tsp olive oil
- To taste, add salt and pepper.
- Different vegetable sticks (cucumbers, bell peppers, and carrots) for dipping

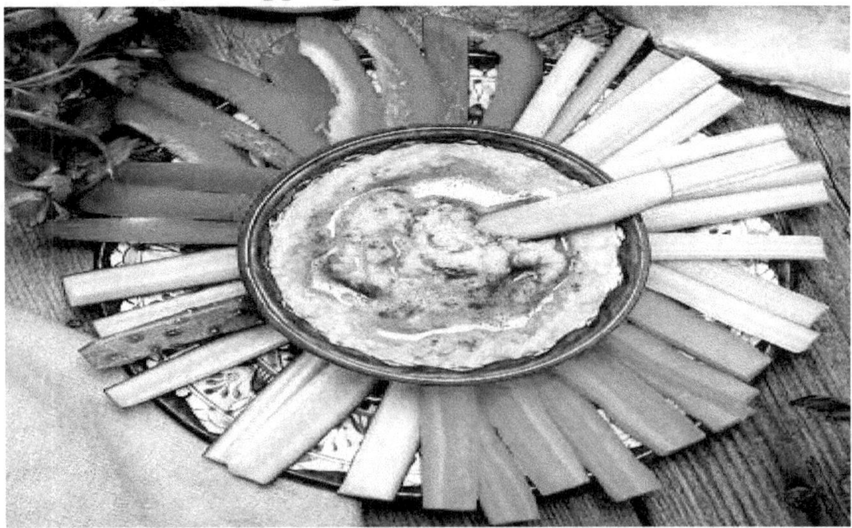

Method:

1. In a food processor, combine the chickpeas, garlic, tahini, lemon juice, olive oil, salt, and pepper.
2. Blend until smooth and creamy, adding more olive oil or water as needed to get the desired consistency.
3. Serve the veggie sticks with roasted red pepper hummus as a satisfying and healthful snack option.

2. <u>Banana Bites with Almond Butter</u>

15 minutes for preparation

Components:

- Two fully ripe bananas
- Butter with almonds
- Chia seeds
- Almond slices
- Honey (not required)

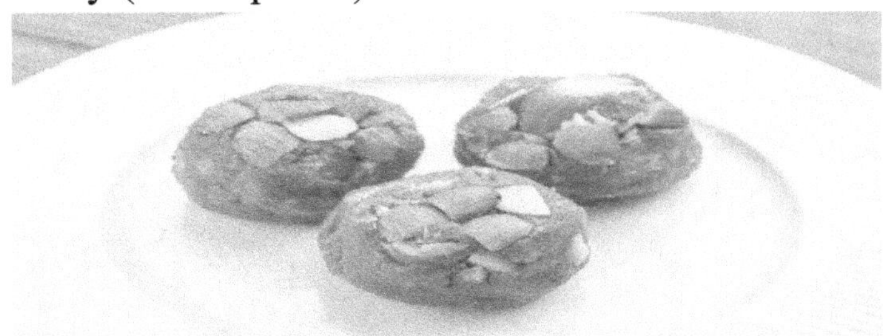

Technique:

1. Slice the bananas into little pieces after peeling.
2. Spread each and every banana slice with almond butter.
3. Add sliced almonds and chia seeds as garnish.
4. Drizzle with honey if desired for a touch of sweetness.
5. Enjoy these bite-sized almond butter bananas as a quick and satisfying snack while you're pregnant.

3. <u>Dark Chocolate Avocado Mousse</u>

Thirty minutes for preparation

Components:

- A pair of mature avocados
- 1/4 cup powdered cocoa
- 1/4 cup honey or maple syrup
- One tsp of vanilla extract
- A dash of salt
- Dark chocolate shavings (optional) as a garnish

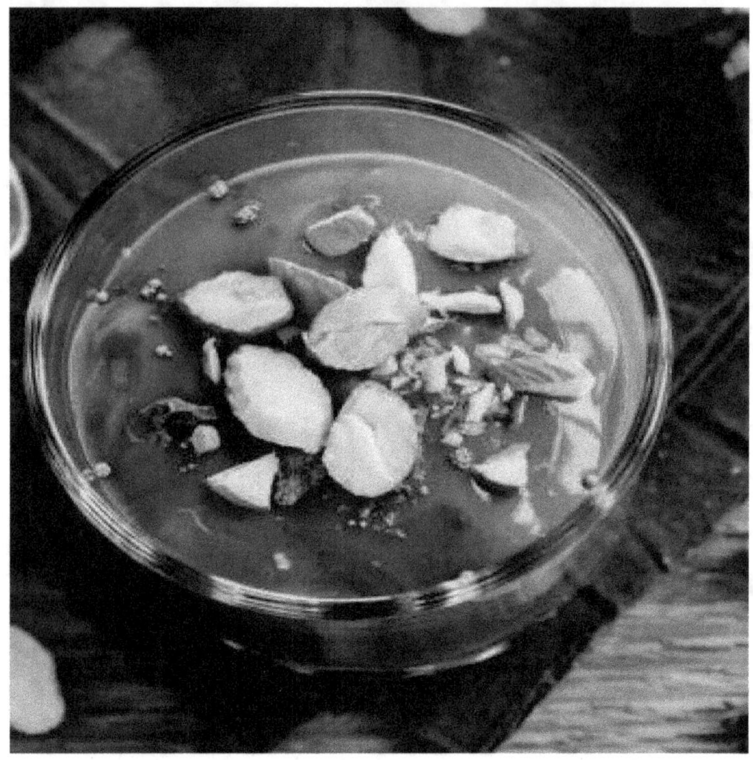

Technique:

1. Fill a food processor with the avocado flesh.
2. Add the cocoa powder, vanilla extract, salt, and honey or maple syrup.
3. Blend until smooth and creamy, scraping down the sides as needed.
4. Spoon dark chocolate-covered avocado mousse onto serving dishes.
5. You may add dark chocolate shavings as a garnish if you'd like.

6. Allow the meal to chill in the refrigerator for at least 20 minutes before serving.
7. Indulge in the decadent and nourishing chocolate avocado mousse without feeling bad.

4. <u>Mediterranean Yogurt Parfait with Fresh Berries</u>

15 minutes for preparation

Components:

- Yogurt with Greek flavor
- Fresh berries, such as raspberries, blueberries, and strawberries
- Cereal
- Optional: honey or maple syrup

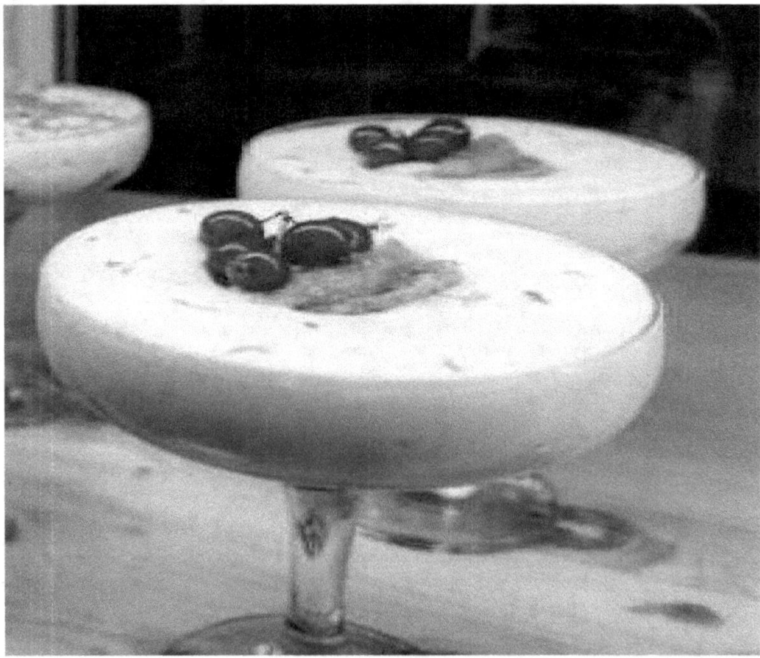

Technique:

1. Fill a glass or plate with Greek yogurt, granola, and fresh berries.
2. For added sweetness, if desired, sprinkle with honey or maple syrup.
3. Keep adding layers until the glass or bowl is filled.
4. Add extra berries and granola to the top for crunch.
5. Treat yourself to this tasty and nutrient-dense Mediterranean yogurt parfait for a snack.

5. <u>Almond-stuffed dates with a Mediterranean flavor</u>

Ten minutes for preparation

Components:

- Pitted Medjool dates
- Almonds
- Goat or cream cheese (optional)
- Honey (not required)

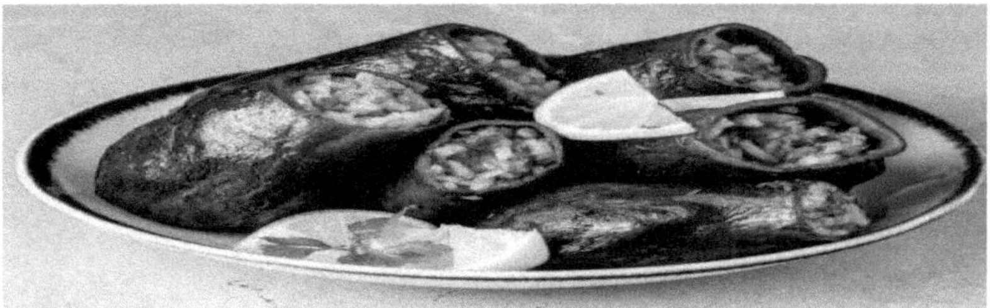

Method:

1. Insert an almond or almond butter into the center of each pitted date.
2. For an even more opulent twist, dab each date with cream cheese or goat cheese.
3. Drizzle some honey on top for a touch of sweetness.
4. Serve these Mediterranean-stuffed dates as a satisfying and stimulating snack while expecting a baby.

6. <u>Greek Feta and Olive Tapenade on Whole Grain Crackers</u>

15 minutes for preparation

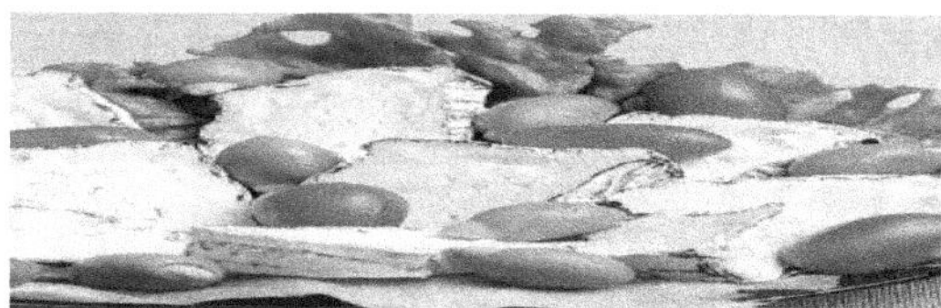

Components:

- Crushed Feta cheese
- Pitted and chopped Kalamata olives
- Chopped sun-dried tomatoes
- Chopped fresh parsley
- Zest of lemon
- Whole grain crackers

Technique:

1. In a bowl, mix the lemon zest, chopped olives, sun-dried tomatoes, parsley, and crumbled feta cheese.
2. Add feta and olive tapenade on the top of the whole grain crackers.
3. Add additional parsley or lemon zest as a garnish if you'd like.
4. Indulge in this delightful Greek-inspired snack that combines creamy feta, salty olives, and sour sun-dried tomatoes.

7. <u>Nuts and Dried Fruit in Mediterranean Trail Mix</u>

Ten minutes for preparation

Components:

- Almonds
- Walnuts
- Pistachios
- Chopped dried apricots
- Cut up dried figs
- Dried cranberries or raisins

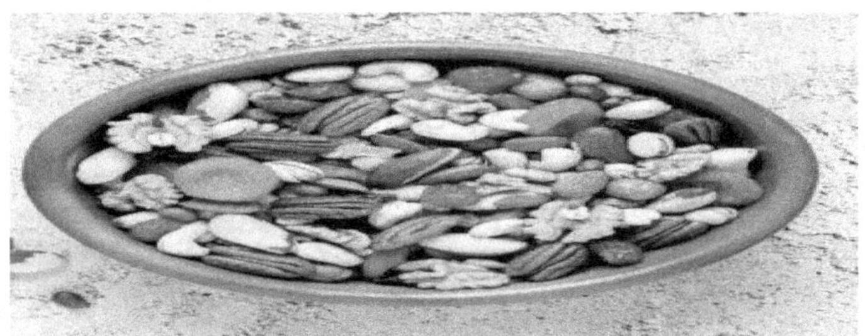

Technique:

1. Arrange the almonds, walnuts, pistachios, raisins or dried cranberries, dried figs, and dried apricots on a plate.
2. To make the trail mix portable for eating on the go, divide it into small bags or containers.
   3. Enjoy this Mediterranean-inspired, high-nutrient trail mix as a satisfying snack when pregnant.

8. <u>Mango Puree with Mediterranean Chia Seed Pudding</u>

Twenty minutes of prep time

Components:

For the pudding with chia seeds:

- Chia seeds
- Coconut or almond milk
- Honey or maple syrup

Regarding the pureed mango:

- Diced and peeled ripe mango - Lemon juice
- Honey or coconut sugar (optional)

Technique:

For the pudding with chia seeds:

1.   In a bowl, mix the chia seeds, honey, maple syrup, and almond or coconut milk.
2.   Cover and refrigerate the chia seeds overnight to allow them to thicken.

About the mango puree:

3.   In a blender, combine the diced mango, lemon juice, honey, or coconut sugar; mix until smooth.

4.   Spoon the chia seed pudding and mango puree into serving glasses.

5.   Allow the meal to chill in the refrigerator for at least 20 minutes before serving.

6.   Enjoy this rich, creamy, and delectable Mediterranean chia seed pudding as a fantastic post-dinner snack.

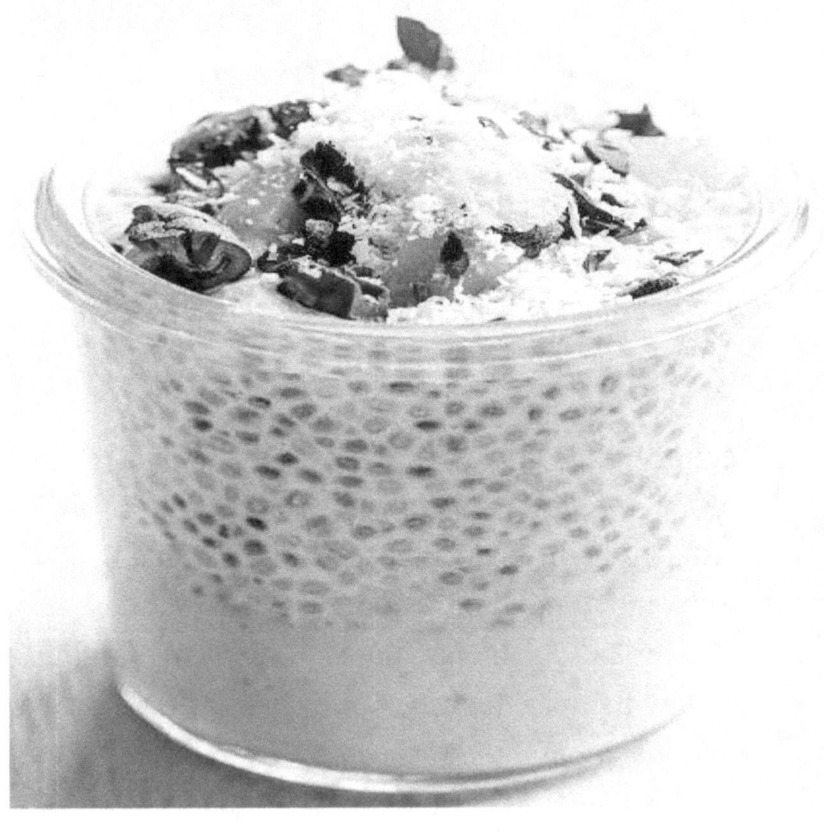

9. <u>Roasted Chickpeas with Herbs & Spices from the Mediterranean</u>

40 minutes for preparation

Ingredients: -

- Drained and washed canned chickpeas
- Olive oil
- Smoked paprika
- Cumin
- Powdered garlic
- Pepper and salt

Technique:

1. Set the oven's temperature to 400°F.
2. In a bowl, combine the chickpeas, salt, pepper, cumin, smoked paprika, and garlic powder.
3. Arrange the seasoned chickpeas on a parchment paper-lined baking sheet.
4. Roast for 30 to 35 minutes, or until crispy and browned.
5. After roasting, let the chickpeas cool down and enjoy a crispy, high-protein snack.

10. <u>Honey-Lemon Salad with Mediterranean Fruits</u>

20 minutes of preparation time

Ingredients: -

1.A variety of fresh fruits (grapes, melon, and berries)
2.Finely chopped mint leaves (optional)

Regarding the lemon-honey dressing:
Juice from lemons and honey

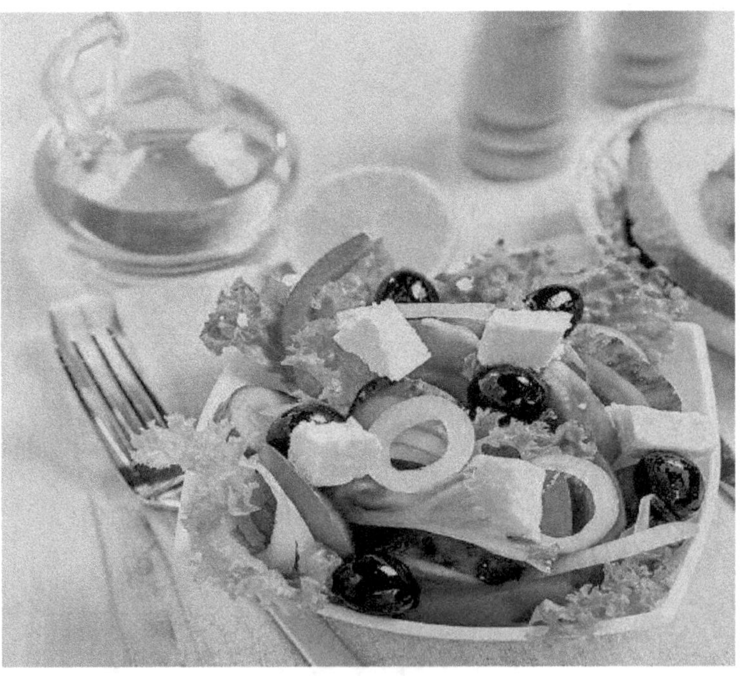

Technique:

1. Cut the fresh fruit into bite-sized pieces and transfer it to a plate.
2. In a separate bowl, combine the honey and lemon juice to make the dressing.
3. Drizzle a honey-lemon dressing over the fruit salad and toss lightly to coat.
4. Garnish with finely chopped mint leaves, if desired.
5. Present this vibrant and refreshing Mediterranean fruit salad as a light and hydrated snack.

11. <u>Almond and Honey Greek Yogurt Parfait</u>

Ten minutes for preparation

Yogurt with Greek flavor

Ingredients:
1. Honey
2. Chopped almonds

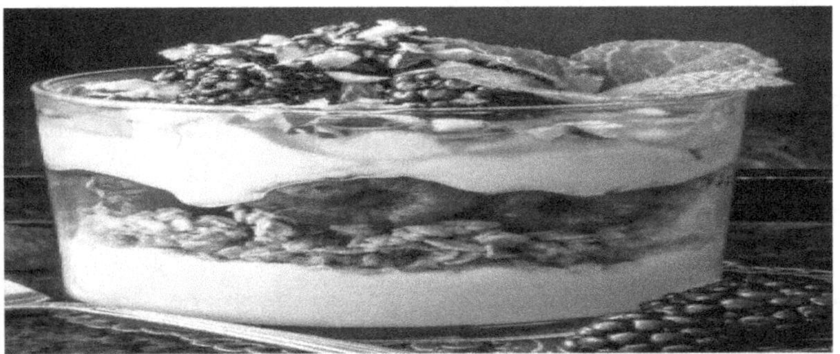

Method:

1. Place Greek yogurt, honey, and chopped almonds in a bowl.
2. To get the required thickness, repeat the layers.

3. Savor this filling and creamy Greek yogurt parfait as a healthy after-meal.

12. <u>Feta and cherry tomato salad with Mediterranean quinoa</u>

Twenty minutes for preparation
Ingredients:

- Cooked quinoa;
- Crumbled Feta cheese;
- Halved cherry tomatoes;
- Chopped fresh parsley; lemon juice
- Olive oil

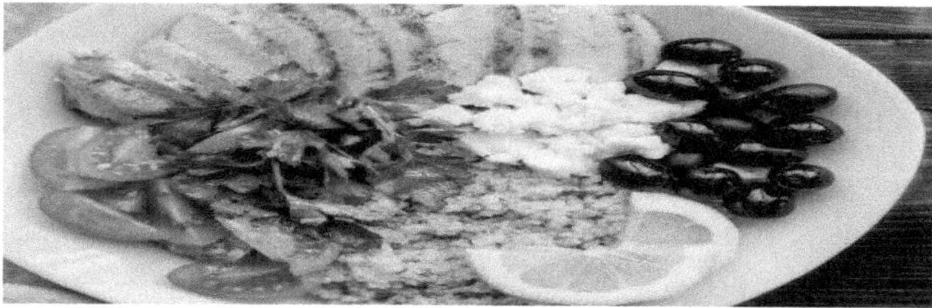

Technique:

1. Combine the cooked quinoa, olive oil, lemon juice, feta cheese, cherry tomatoes, and parsley in a bowl.
2. Add salt and pepper to taste and toss again to

thoroughly combine.

3. Serve this savory and light snack, a refreshing Mediterranean quinoa salad.

13. <u>Pita chips paired with roasted eggplant dip</u>

30 minutes for preparation;

- ➢ Ingredients:
- ➢ Eggplant
- ➢ Lemon juice
- ➢ Cloves of garlic
- ➢ Pita bread (cut into wedges for dipping)
- ➢ Olive oil - Tahini

Technique:

1. Roast eggplant until it becomes blackened and tender.

2. Remove the eggplant's peel and puree the meat until smooth, adding garlic, lemon juice, tahini, and olive oil.

3. Present the roasted eggplant dip with pita chips to create a flavorful and filling appetizer.

14. <u>Mint-infused Watermelon Feta Salad</u>

Prepare in 15 minutes using the following

Ingredients: -

➢ Cubed watermelon
➢ Crumbled Feta cheese
➢ Chop fresh mint leaves
➢ Balsamic glaze (not required)

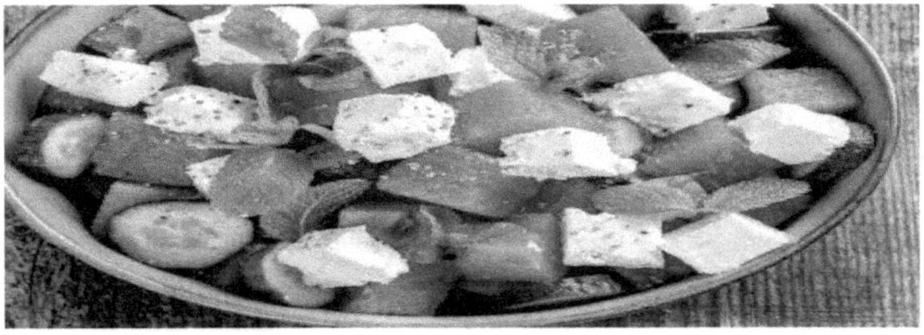

Technique:
1. Combine chopped mint leaves, crumbled feta cheese, and watermelon cubes in a bowl.
2. For extra taste, drizzle with balsamic glaze if preferred.
3. Savor this tasty and hydrating watermelon feta salad as a light snack.

15. <u>Cucumber-Dill Mediterranean Chickpea Salad</u>

15 minutes for preparation

Ingredients:

- Drained and rinsed canned chickpeas;
- Sliced cucumber;
- finely chopped red onion;
- chopped fresh dill; and lemon juice
- Olive oil

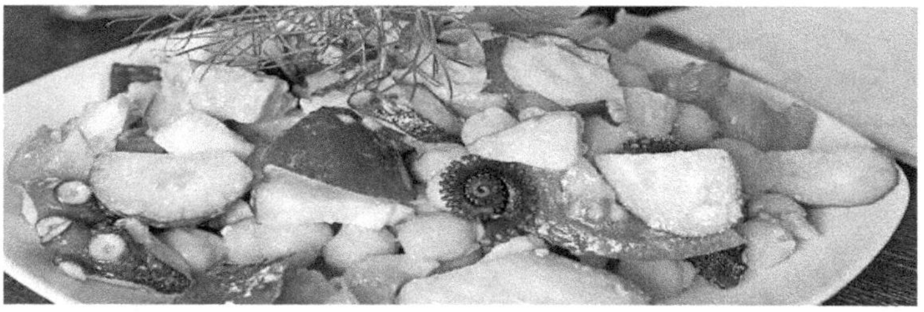

Technique:

1. In a bowl, combine the chickpeas, lemon juice, olive oil, cucumber, red onion, and dill.
2. Combine by tossing, then season to taste with salt and pepper.
3. Present this flavorful Mediterranean chickpea salad

as a high-protein snack choice.

16. <u>Stuffed Mushrooms with Feta and Spinach</u>

Twenty-five minutes for preparation

Ingredients:
- Chopped spinach,
- Crumbled Feta cheese,
- Large mushrooms with stems removed,
- A minced garlic
- Olive oil

Technique:
1. Set the oven's temperature to 375°F.
2. Sauté garlic and spinach in olive oil in a pan until the spinach wilts.
3. Stuff spinach mixture into mushrooms; sprinkle feta cheese crumbles on top.
4. Bake the mushrooms for 15 to 20 minutes, or until they are soft.
5. Savor these stuffed mushrooms with feta and spinach as a tasty snack.

17. <u>Pita bread and Mediterranean Tzatziki</u>

15 minutes for preparation;
Ingredients:

- Greek yogurt
- Drained and shredded cucumber
- Minced garlic
- Lemon juice
- Chopped fresh dill
- Toasty pita bread for dipping

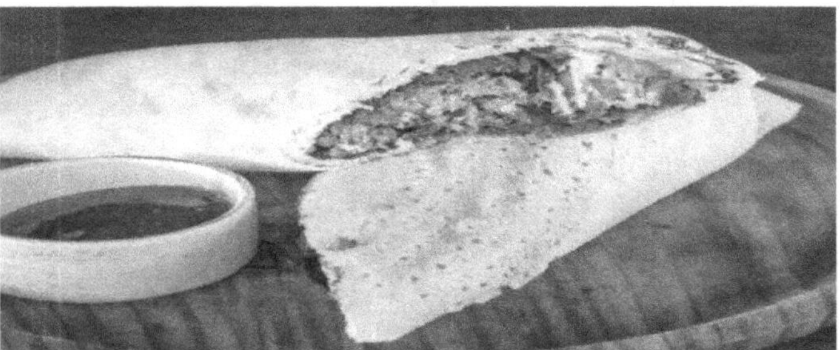

Technique:
1. Combine Greek yogurt, grated cucumber, dill, lemon juice, and garlic in a bowl.
2. To let flavors to merge, chill in the refrigerator for a minimum of half an hour.
3. Toasted pita bread is a nice and delicious snack when paired with tzatziki.

18. <u>Quinoa and Chickpea Stuffed Bell Peppers</u>

40 minutes for preparation

Ingredients:
- ➢ Sliced cherry tomatoes;
- ➢ Drained and rinsed canned chickpeas;
- ➢ Cooked quinoa;
- ➢ Split and deseeded bell peppers;
- ➢ Crumbled feta cheese

Technique:
1. Set the oven's temperature to 375°F.
2. Combine the cooked quinoa, feta cheese, cherry tomatoes, and chickpeas in a bowl.
3. Stuff the quinoa mixture into the bell pepper halves.
4. Bake the peppers for 25 to 30 minutes, or until they are soft.
5. Savor these vibrantly colored filled bell peppers as a filling and healthy after-meal.

19. <u>Cucumber cups with hummus and olives from the Mediterranean</u>

Twenty minutes for preparation

Ingredients: -

➢ Pitted and halved Kalamata olives
➢ Hummus
➢ English cucumbers cut into rounds

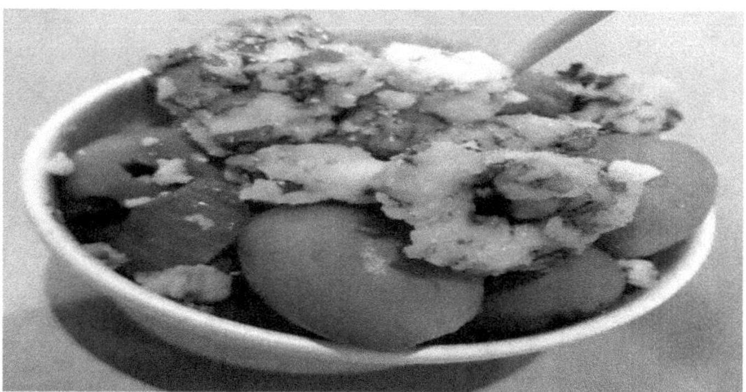

Technique:

1. To make a cup, hollow out the middle of each round of cucumber with a spoon.

2. Spoon hummus into each cucumber cup, then garnish with half of the Kalamata olives.

3. Present these light and energizing Mediterranean

cucumber cups as a snack.

20. Date Energy Balls with Pistachios

Twenty minutes of prep time plus chilling time

Components:

- Pitted dates
- Shelled pistachios
- Coconut flakes
- Butter with almonds

Technique:

1. Process dates, pistachios, coconut flakes, and almond butter in a food processor until the mixture comes together.
2. Form the mixture into tiny balls and refrigerate for a minimum of half an hour.
3. Snacklift on these nutrient-dense pistachio date energy balls for on-the-go bursts of energy.

21. Balsamic-Glazed Mediterranean Caprese Skewers

Prep Time: 15 minutes;

Ingredients:

- Fresh mozzarella balls,
- VCherry tomatoes,
- Basil leaves
- balsamic glaze

Technique:

1. Thread fresh mozzarella balls, cherry tomatoes, and basil leaves onto skewers.

2. Add a balsamic glaze drizzle for more taste and sweetness.

3. As a simple but sophisticated snack option, serve these vibrant Caprese skewers.

22. <u>The Almonds with Rosemary and Lemon</u>

Twenty minutes of prep time (plus baking time)

Components:
- ➢ Almonds
- ➢ Chopped fresh rosemary
- ➢ Lemon zest - Olive oil - Sea salt

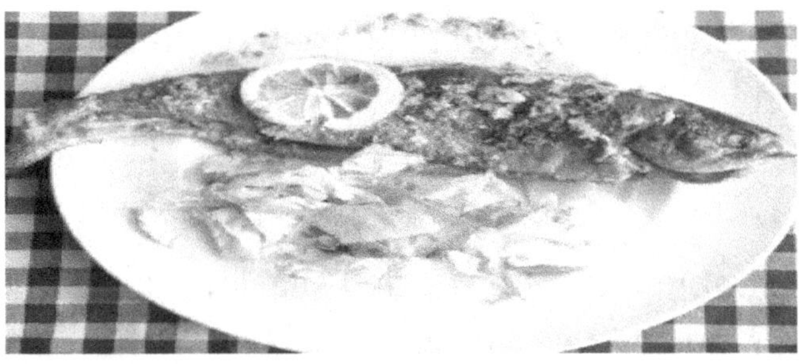

Technique:
1. Set the oven's temperature to 325°F.
2. Combine almonds, rosemary, lemon zest, olive oil, and sea salt in a bowl.
3. Arrange the almonds on a parchment paper-lined baking sheet.
4. Roast for 15 to 20 minutes, or until aromatic and browned.
5. Let the roasted almonds cool down before

savoring them as a flavorful and crispy snack.

23. <u>Mediterranean Rice and Herb Stuffed Grape Leaves (Dolmas)</u>

Forty minutes of prep time plus cooking time

Components:

- ➤ Fresh or preserved grape leaves
- ➤ Cooked Arborio rice
- ➤ Freshly chopped parsley
- ➤ Chopped mint leaves
- ➤ Lemon juice

Technique:

1. To soften fresh grape leaves, blanch them for a brief period of time in boiling water.
2. Combine cooked rice, lemon juice, parsley, and mint leaves in a basin.
3. To make dolmas, take a tablespoon of the rice mixture and wrap it firmly around each grape leaf.
4. Serve these fragrant grape leaves filled with Mediterranean spices as an interesting and

filling snack.

24. <u>Quinoa and spinach stuffed bell pepper rings with a Mediterranean flair</u>

Thirty minutes of prep time (plus baking time)

Components:

> Sliced red or yellow bell peppers into rings
> Prepared quinoa
> Young spinach leaves
> Feta cheese

Technique:

1. Set the oven's temperature to 375°F.

2. Sauté baby spinach in a pan until it wilts.

3. Stuff each ring of bell pepper with cooked quinoa, sautéed spinach, and feta cheese crumbles.

4. Bake the peppers for 20 to 25 minutes, or until they are soft.

5. Snackle on these vibrant filled bell pepper rings for a healthy choice.

25. <u>Berries and Mediterranean Chia Seed Pudding Parfait</u>

Ten minutes for preparation plus chilling time

Components:
For the pudding with chia seeds:
- Chia seeds
- Milk with almonds
- Syrup from maple
Regarding the berry compote:
- A variety of berries, including blueberries and strawberries
- Lemon juice

Technique:

For the pudding with chia seeds:
1. Combine the chia seeds, almond milk, and maple syrup in a bowl.
2. To thicken, chill in the refrigerator for at least four hours or overnight.
Regarding the berry compote:
3. Simmer mixed berries and lemon juice in a saucepan until the berries are tender.
4. Arrange the berry compote and chia seed pudding in

serving cups.

5. Before serving, let the food cool for a further half hour in the refrigerator.

6. Savor this luscious parfait of creamy chia seed pudding and colorful fruit compote as a filling after-meal or snack.

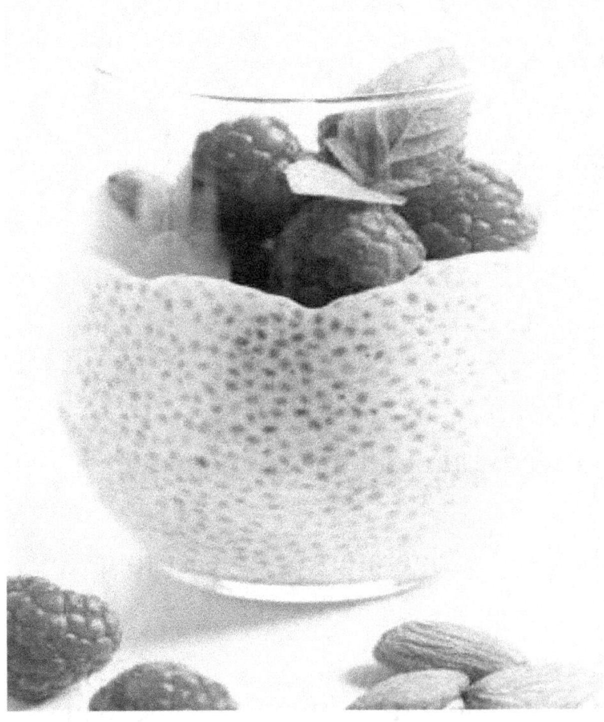

26. <u>Roasted Vegetables and Mediterranean</u> Lentil Salad

Thirty minutes of prep time plus cooking time
Components:
- Lentils
- A variety of veggies, including bell peppers and zucchini; - Red onions
- Cherry tomatoes
Technique:
1. Prepare lentils as directed on the box until they are soft.
2. Roast a variety of veggies in the oven with cherry tomatoes and red onions until they caramelize.
3. In a bowl, combine cooked lentils and roasted veggies.
4. For extra taste, drizzle with balsamic vinegar and olive oil.
5. Present this filling and nutrient-dense Mediterranean lentil salad as a snack.

27. <u>Triangles of Greek Spanakopita</u>

45 minutes for preparation plus baking time

Components:

- ➤ Phyllo bread,
- ➤ feta cheese,
- ➤ spinach, and dill

Technique:

1. Set the oven's temperature to 375°F.
2. In a bowl, combine cooked spinach, crumbled feta cheese, and finely chopped dill.
3. Divide the phyllo dough into strips, then stuff the spinach-feta mixture into each strip.
4. Fold into triangles and arrange on a parchment paper-lined baking pan.
5. Bake for 20 to 25 minutes, or until crispy and golden brown.
6. Savor these crispy pieces of Greek spanakopita as a tasty snack or starter.

28. Mediterranean Roasted Red Pepper Tapenade Crostini

30-minute prep plus baking time

Components:

About the tapenade of roasted red pepper:

- Red pepper flakes

- Olives Kalamata

- Garlic

Regarding the crostini:

- Slices of baguette

- Olive oil

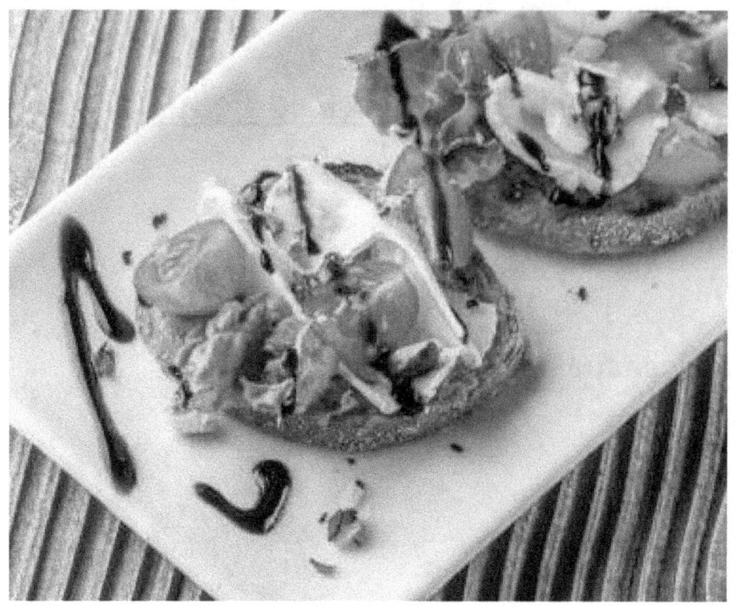

Technique:

About the tapenade of roasted red pepper:

1. In a food processor, blend garlic, Kalamata olives, and roasted red peppers until smooth.

Regarding the crostini:

2. Toasted baguette slices in the oven till golden brown after brushing them with olive oil.

3. Spread roasted red pepper tapenade on top of each crostini.

4. As a sophisticated snack or starter, serve these flavorful Mediterranean roasted red pepper tapenade crostini.

29. <u>Honey-Lime Honey-Skewers with Mediterranean Fruits</u>

Twenty minutes for preparation

Components:

- ➢ Various fresh fruits (strawberries, pineapple pieces, etc.)
- ➢ Lime juice with honey
- ➢ Mint leaves (not required)

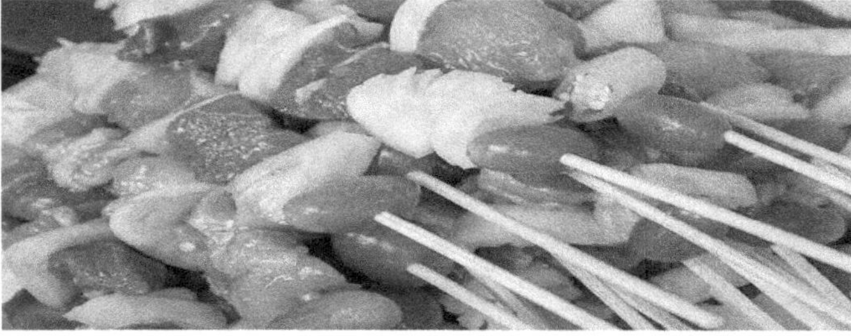

Technique:

1. Thread selected combinations of fresh fruit pieces onto skewers.

2. Drizzle with a combination of honey and lime juice (honey-lime).

3. For extra freshness, garnish with mint leaves if preferred.

4. Serve these bright and delicious
Mediterranean fruit skewers as a snack.

30. <u>Quinoa salad with stuffed avocado halves from the Mediterranean</u>

Thirty minutes for preparation

Ingredients:

- Pitted and halved avocados
- Quinoa salad cooked (quinoa combined with chopped veggies)
- Crumbled feta cheese
- Chopped fresh parsley
  slices of lemon as a garnish

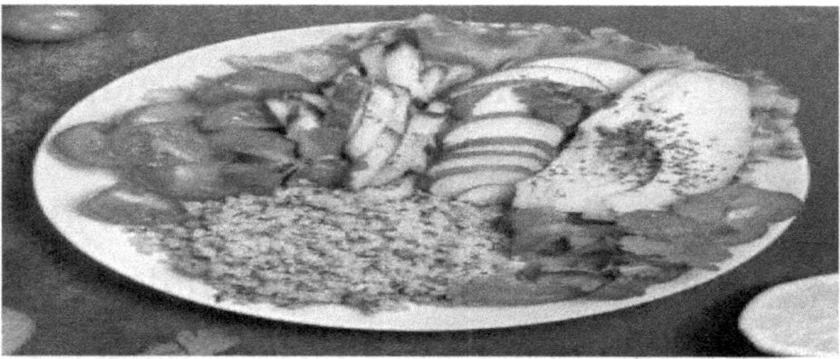

Technique:

1. Spoon cooked quinoa salad mixture into each avocado half; garnish with parsley and crumbled feta cheese.

2. Present packed avocado halves with a lemon juice drizzle.
3. Savor these rich, creamy Mediterranean-stuffed avocado halves as a filling after-school treat or as a light dinner.

These snacks and sweets are not only delicious but also nutrient-rich, which can help you stay healthy during your pregnancy. Whether you're craving something spicy like roasted red pepper hummus or something sweet like dark chocolate avocado mousse, these recipes provide the ideal balance of flavors and textures to satisfy your cravings and nourish your growing child's body. Incorporate these Mediterranean-inspired items into your regular diet for a joyful and healthful pregnancy.
Remember to talk to your doctor about any dietary restrictions or adjustments to ensure you are obtaining the nutrients you especially need during pregnancy.

Enjoy these guilt-free treats and snacks while you enjoy the joys of pregnancy and nourish yourself with nutritious ingredients from Mediterranean cuisine.

Have fun in the kitchen!

CHAPTER SEVEN

Tips for Eating Out and Traveling While Pregnant

Expectant mothers may have particular difficulties while dining out and traveling, but it is still feasible to keep a healthy, balanced diet even when traveling if you plan ahead and make thoughtful decisions. This chapter will discuss ways to promote a healthy pregnancy while traveling, such as packing nutrient-dense snacks and making smart restaurant selections.

Selecting Healthful Menu Items at Restaurants

It's crucial to prioritize meals high in vital nutrients while eating out while pregnant while avoiding possible hazards like foodborne infections. Here are some pointers to help you choose healthfully while dining out:

1. Make A Wise Choice: Seek for eateries that provide a range of healthful and fresh selections, such salads, grilled meats, and whole grains. To make sure you are receiving a decent mix of vitamins and minerals, choose meals that contain a lot of fruits and vegetables.

2. Pay Attention to Portion proportions:

Although being pregnant could make you more hungry, it's crucial to pay attention to portion proportions to prevent overindulging. If you are eating with someone, think about splitting the dish or asking for a half portion if it is available.

3. Steer Clear of Raw or Undercooked

Foods: It's better to stay away from raw or undercooked meats, shellfish, eggs, and unpasteurized dairy products to lower your chance of contracting a foodborne disease. For food safety, use completely cooked choices.

4. Reduce salt and Added Sugars: Meals at

restaurants are often heavy in added sugars and salt, which may aggravate pregnancy-related bloating and diabetes. Pick foods with less salt and stay away from sugary drinks in favor of water or unsweetened liquids.

5. Personalize Your Order: Don't hesitate to

request changes to accommodate certain dietary requirements. Choose grilled or steamed items over fried ones, ask for dressings and sauces on the side, and choose healthier sides like a side salad or steamed veggies.

6. Listen to Your Body: When eating out, pay attention to your body's signals of hunger and fullness. To avoid overindulging, eat gently and quit when you're full.

How to Bring Healthful Snacks on Trip

While traveling while pregnant may be thrilling, it's important to prepare ahead of time and bring wholesome foods to keep you feeling full and active. Here are some suggestions for bringing healthy snacks on trips:

1. **Fresh Fruits and Vegetables**: For a fast and simple snack that is high in fiber and vitamins, pack portable alternatives like apples, bananas, baby carrots, or cherry tomatoes.

2. **Nuts and Seeds:** A great source of protein, healthy fats, and vital nutrients include almonds, walnuts, pumpkin seeds, and sunflower seeds. Make your own trail mix, or measure it out into individual servings for a filling snack.

3. **Greek Yogurt Cups:** A portable, high-protein snack that might help you feel content and full while traveling are pre-portioned Greek yogurt cups.

4. **Whole Grain Crackers with Nut Butter:** When combined with peanut butter or almond butter, whole grain crackers provide a well-balanced source of

healthy fats, protein, and carbs for long-lasting energy.

5. Homemade Energy Bars: To make a nutrient-dense snack that is portable, make your own energy bars using components like oats, almonds, dried fruits, and seeds.

6. Hummus with Veggie Sticks: For a cool and high-fiber snack alternative, package individual hummus containers with sliced bell peppers, cucumbers, or celery sticks.

7. Dried Fruit and Nut Mix: For a delightful combination of sweetness and crunch, make your own mix of dried fruits (like apricots, cranberries, or raisins) and nuts (like cashews, pistachios, or pecans).

8. Hard-Boiled Eggs: Made ahead of time and consumed as a travel-friendly snack, hard-boiled eggs are a handy source of protein and minerals.

9. Rice Cakes with Avocado: For a filling and light snack that offers fiber, healthy fats, and vital nutrients, spread mashed avocado on rice cakes.

10. Hydration Essentials: To keep hydrated on your trip, don't forget to bring a reusable water bottle. For a cool variation, try adding some taste with cucumber or lemon slices.

Making advance plans and bringing wholesome snacks with you on the road can guarantee that you always have access to wholesome alternatives. These snacks will not only help you stay healthy throughout your pregnancy, but they will also provide your developing baby the vital nutrition it needs.

To promote a healthy and nutritious pregnant experience, don't forget to pay attention to your body's hunger signals, remain hydrated, and make thoughtful decisions whether eating out or traveling.

We'll talk about the value of self-care throughout pregnancy and how to put your physical and mental health first as you get ready to become a mother in the next chapter.

Happy munching and safe travels!

CHAPTER EIGHT

The Value of Taking Care of Oneself While Pregnant

Maintaining your physical and mental well-being during pregnancy is crucial as you get ready to become a mother. Taking care of yourself helps your child grow normally and benefits you as well. This chapter will discuss the value of self-care throughout pregnancy and provide doable methods for putting your mental and physical well-being first.

Physical Self-Surveillance

1. Regular Exercise: Maintaining an active lifestyle throughout pregnancy helps enhance general wellbeing, lower stress levels, and improve circulation. Prenatal yoga, swimming, or walking are examples of low-impact workouts that may help you stay fit and encourage a healthy pregnancy.

2. Balanced Nutrition: It's important to provide your

kid with the nutrients they need to support their growth and development by eating a well-rounded diet full of fruits, vegetables, whole grains, lean proteins, and healthy fats. To make sure you are getting the nutrients you need throughout pregnancy, speak with your doctor or a qualified dietitian.

3. Sufficient Rest: During pregnancy, getting adequate sleep is essential for your physical well-being and level of vitality. To battle weariness, aim for 7-9 hours of excellent sleep each night and think about taking short naps throughout the day.

4. Prenatal Care: Keep all of your prenatal visits and heed your doctor's advice for prenatal exams, screenings, and immunizations. To ensure a safe pregnancy and to track your baby's progress, regular check-ups are crucial.

5. Hydration: To maintain optimum body functioning and keep hydrated, sip plenty of water throughout the day. Make it a point to drink enough water each day since dehydration might cause difficulties during pregnancy.

Mental Well-Being

1. Stress management: There are many different feelings that may accompany pregnancy, from enthusiasm to worry. To control tension and encourage relaxation, use stress-reduction methods like deep breathing, mindfulness, meditation, or light exercise.

2. Self-Compassion: Throughout your pregnancy, treat yourself with kindness and cultivate self-compassion. Recognize that feeling a range of emotions is natural and allow yourself to put your health first.

3. Support System: During your pregnant experience, surround yourself with a network of family, friends, or medical professionals who can give emotional support, advice, and encouragement. Never be afraid to ask for assistance when you need it.

4. Mindfulness and Relaxation: To encourage relaxation and lessen anxiety, include mindfulness exercises into your daily routine, such as meditation, visualization, or light stretching. Engaging in self-care practices may foster a stronger bond between you and your body and child.

5. Mental Health Check-Ins: Keep an eye on your mental well-being throughout your pregnancy and get treatment from a specialist if you exhibit signs of anxiety, depression, or other mental health issues. During this period of transition, your mental and physical health are equally vital.

6. Pampering Treatments: To nourish your body and encourage relaxation, treat yourself to self-care rituals like warm baths, mild skincare regimens, or prenatal massages. During pregnancy, giving yourself some TLC may help you feel refreshed and taken care of.

Recall that taking care of oneself is not selfish; rather, it is essential to preserving a good pregnancy and being ready for parenthood. You are fostering a strong bond with your unborn child and laying the groundwork for a happy pregnancy experience by putting your physical and mental health first.

We will look at postpartum self-care techniques in the last chapter of this book to help you heal and get used to life with a baby. Watch this space for helpful advice on taking care of yourself after giving birth.

Embrace yourself, soon-to-be mother!

CHAPTER NINE

BONUSES

Quinoa and Chickpea Salad with Lemon-Tahini Dressing

Prep Time: 20 minutes

Ingredients:

- 1 cup cooked quinoa

- 1 can chickpeas, drained and rinsed

- 1/2 cup cherry tomatoes, halved

- 1/4 cup red onion, finely chopped

- 1/4 cup fresh parsley, chopped

- 1/4 cup feta cheese, crumbled (optional)

- Salt and pepper to taste

For the Lemon-Tahini Dressing:

- 2 tablespoons tahini

- 2 tablespoons lemon juice

- 1 tablespoon olive oil

- 1 clove garlic, minced

- 1/2 teaspoon honey (optional)

- Water to thin out the dressing

- Salt and pepper to taste

Method:

1. In a large mixing bowl, combine the cooked quinoa, chickpeas, cherry tomatoes, red onion, and parsley. Toss to mix well.

2. In a small bowl, whisk together the tahini, lemon juice, olive oil, garlic, honey (if using), salt, and pepper. Add water gradually to achieve your desired consistency for the dressing.

3. Pour the Lemon-Tahini Dressing over the quinoa and chickpea mixture. Toss until everything is well coated.

4. Taste and adjust seasoning if needed. Add more salt and pepper as desired.

5. Sprinkle crumbled feta cheese over the salad if using.

6. Serve immediately or refrigerate for later. Enjoy this nutritious and flavorful Quinoa and Chickpea Salad with Lemon-Tahini Dressing!

Grilled Vegetable Wrap with Hummus

Prep Time: 30 minutes

Ingredients:

- 1 zucchini, sliced lengthwise

- 1 yellow bell pepper, sliced

- 1 red onion, sliced

- 1 tablespoon olive oil

- Salt and pepper to taste

- 4 whole wheat wraps or tortillas

- 1 cup hummus

- Fresh parsley or cilantro for garnish (optional)

Method:

1. Preheat a grill pan or outdoor grill over medium-high heat.

2. In a bowl, toss the zucchini, bell pepper, and red onion slices with olive oil, salt, and pepper until well coated.

3. Grill the vegetables for about 5-7 minutes on each side, or until they are tender and have nice grill marks.

4. Warm the whole wheat wraps or tortillas in a microwave or on a skillet for a few seconds to make them pliable.

5. Spread a generous layer of hummus onto each wrap.

6. Place a portion of the grilled vegetables in the center of each wrap.

7. Sprinkle fresh parsley or cilantro over the vegetables for added freshness (if using).

8. Fold in the sides of the wrap and roll it up tightly.

9. Cut the wraps in half diagonally and serve immediately.

Enjoy this delicious and nutritious Grilled Vegetable Wrap with Hummus, perfect for expecting moms looking for a Mediterranean-inspired meal option!

Mediterranean Lentil Soup with Spinach

Prep Time: 45 minutes

Ingredients:

- 1 cup dried green or brown lentils, rinsed and drained

- 1 onion, diced

- 2 cloves garlic, minced

- 1 carrot, diced

- 1 celery stalk, diced

- 1 can (14 oz) diced tomatoes

- 4 cups vegetable broth

- 1 teaspoon ground cumin

- 1 teaspoon ground coriander

- 1/2 teaspoon smoked paprika

- Salt and pepper to taste

- 2 cups fresh spinach, chopped

- Juice of 1 lemon

- Fresh parsley or cilantro for garnish (optional)

Method:

1. In a large pot, heat a little bit of olive oil over medium heat. Add the diced onion, garlic, carrot, and celery. Cook until vegetables are softened, about 5 minutes.

2. Add the lentils, diced tomatoes (with their juices), vegetable broth, cumin, coriander, smoked paprika, salt, and pepper to the pot. Stir to combine.

3. Bring the soup to a boil, then reduce heat to low and let it simmer for about 30-35 minutes, or until the lentils are tender.

4. Stir in the chopped spinach and lemon juice. Cook for an additional 5 minutes until the spinach is wilted.

5. Taste and adjust seasoning if needed.

6. Ladle the Mediterranean Lentil Soup with Spinach into bowls and garnish with fresh parsley or cilantro if desired.

7. Serve hot and enjoy the comforting flavors of this nutritious soup.

This Mediterranean Lentil Soup with Spinach is packed with protein, fiber, and vitamins, making it a perfect addition to your Mediterranean-inspired meal plan for expecting moms.

Strategies for Postpartum Self-Care

Best wishes on the birth of your little one! During the postpartum phase, you undergo notable physical and psychological transformations as you recuperate from giving birth and become used to living with a baby. Making self-care a priority during this period is essential to assisting with your recovery, wellbeing, and transition to parenthood. We will look at postpartum self-care techniques in this chapter to help you get through this time of transition with strength and grace.

Physical Self-Surveillance

1. Rest and Recovery: In the first postpartum weeks, pay attention to your body and give rest top priority. Give yourself time to recover following giving birth, sleep as much as you can, and accept assistance from loved ones with domestic chores and kid care.

2. Nutrition and Hydration: To help with your recuperation and energy levels, keep a well-balanced diet full of foods high in nutrients. Drink plenty of

water to stay hydrated throughout the day, particularly if you are nursing a baby.

3. Mild activity: To aid in both your physical and emotional healing, gradually resume mild activity, such as postpartum yoga or walking. Be sure to speak with your doctor before beginning any fitness regimen.

4. Pelvic Floor Care: To strengthen your pelvic floor muscles and promote bladder control and postpartum recovery, do pelvic floor exercises, sometimes referred to as Kegels. For individualized advice, think about seeing a pelvic floor physical therapist.

5. Self-Care Products: To enhance your comfort and recuperation during the postpartum phase, make an investment in postpartum necessities including cozy apparel, nursing bras, perineal care products, and nursing equipment.

Mental Well-Being

1. Emotional Support: During the postpartum phase, rely on your spouse, family, friends, or a support group for emotional support and direction. To reduce

emotions of overload or isolation, be open and honest about your experiences and feelings.

2. Mental Health Check-Ins: Keep a careful eye on your mental well-being and get treatment from a professional if you exhibit any signs of anxiety, sadness, or other mood problems after giving birth. Taking care of your mental health is crucial to taking care of both you and your child.

3. Self-Compassion: When navigating the difficulties of being a new mother, treat yourself with kindness. Put your own needs first and give yourself compassion and understanding as you learn to cope with the responsibilities of taking care of a baby.

4. Time for You: Schedule little, daily periods of self-care, even if they are just for a few minutes. Go for a stroll, read a book, have a soothing bath, or indulge in a pastime that makes you happy and relaxed.

5. Connection with Baby: Make skin-to-skin contact, cuddle, converse, sing, and make eye contact with your infant to strengthen your link. These exchanges foster emotions of intimacy and connection in addition to being good for your baby's growth.

6. Professional Support: If you need extra assistance with mental struggles, nursing issues, or adapting to parenting, think about seeing a therapist, counselor, or lactation consultant. Expert assistance may provide insightful advice and helpful coping mechanisms for adjusting to postpartum changes.

Keep in mind that self-care is a continuous habit that changes as you experience the rewards and difficulties of parenting. Making time for your physical and mental health during the postpartum phase can provide the groundwork for a speedy recovery and a happy transition to life with your baby.

As a new mother, acknowledge your courage and fortitude and never forget that you deserve kindness and support throughout this life-changing period. Accept the path ahead with love, tolerance, and self-nurturing.

I'm hoping your postpartum journey brings you health and pleasure!

Foods to Eat if You Want to Boost Fertility

1. Leafy Green Vegetables: High in folate, iron, and other vital elements that promote fertility and general health, leafy green vegetables include spinach, kale, Swiss chard, and others.

2. Berries: Packed with antioxidants, berries such as blueberries, strawberries, raspberries, and blackberries aid in cell damage prevention and enhance reproductive health.

3. Nuts and Seeds: Rich sources of protein, healthy fats, and vital nutrients that help increase fertility include almonds, walnuts, chia seeds, flaxseeds, and pumpkin seeds.

4. Whole Grains: Whole grains, which include quinoa, brown rice, oats, and barley, are rich in fiber, vitamins, and minerals as well as complex carbs that assist hormonal balance and blood sugar regulation.

5. Lean Proteins: To promote egg production and general reproductive health, include lean protein sources in your diet, such as chicken, turkey, fish, tofu, tempeh, and lentils.

6. Dairy Products: To get calcium, protein, and other vital nutrients that boost fertility, choose low-fat or non-fat dairy products such milk, yogurt, and cheese.

7. Avocado: Rich in fiber, antioxidants, vitamins, minerals, and healthy fats, avocados help promote reproductive health and hormonal balance.

8. Citrus Fruits: Vitamin C, folate, and other nutrients that promote fertility and general health are abundant in oranges, grapefruits, lemons, and limes.

It's important to consume lots of water throughout the day to keep hydrated in addition to include these nutrient-rich items in your diet. Reducing the amount of processed meals that are heavy in harmful fats and added sugars will also help you become more fertile and prime your body for a successful birth.

As you get ready for pregnancy, you may boost your fertility and general health by concentrating on a balanced diet that consists of a range of nutrient-rich foods from all food categories. In order to be sure you're fulfilling your unique nutritional requirements and making healthy decisions for both you and your unborn child, don't forget to speak with your healthcare practitioner or a qualified dietitian.

HAVE FUN IN THE KITCHEN!